A colour atlas of
ORAL MEDICINE

Copyright © William R. Tyldesley, 1978
Published by Wolfe Medical Publications Ltd, 1978
Printed in Italy by Staderini S.p.A.
ISBN 7234 0729 0
2nd impression 1981

This book is one of the titles in the series of
Wolfe Medical Atlases, a series which brings
together probably the world's largest systematic
published collection of diagnostic colour
photographs.
For a full list of Atlases in the series, plus
forthcoming titles and details of our surgical,
dental and veterinary Atlases, please write to
Wolfe Medical Publications Ltd, Wolfe House,
3 Conway Street, London W1P 6HE

A COLOUR ATLAS OF
ORAL MEDICINE

WILLIAM R. TYLDESLEY

DDS., Ph.D., FDSRCS.,

Acting Head of Department of Dental Surgery
University of Liverpool

WOLFE MEDICAL PUBLICATIONS LTD

Photography and Acknowledgments

The majority of the patients illustrated were photographed by the author using Kodachrome IIA film, an Exa 500 camera body with a 100mm lens and a Minicam ring flash.

Grateful acknowledgments are made to a number of colleagues who have kindly loaned illustrations of their patients. A few of the illustrations have previously appeared elsewhere, usually in a black-and-white version, and acknowledgments are made to the editors of the journals mentioned for their kind permission to reproduce these. My thanks to: Mr P F Bradley, Mr J C Cooper, Dr P Dufton, Professor E D Farmer, Mr L D Finch, Mr D H Goose, Mr H A Priestland, Dr N R Rowell, Dr F W Yates, The Editors of the British Dental Journal, the British Journal of Oral Surgery and the Journal of the Royal College of Surgeons of Edinburgh.

Contents

Introduction

The discipline of oral medicine is concerned with the study and non-surgical treatment of diseases affecting the oral cavity and related structures. Although many forms of disease are included in this wide remit, the predominant interest is in lesions of the oral mucous membrane and these form the basis of most of the illustrations in this atlas.

Oral medicine has in recent years changed from an almost entirely descriptive study to one in which investigational procedures are of great importance. With this change has come recognition that the abnormalities resulting from many generalised disease processes are first seen within the oral cavity and that early diagnosis may follow on from a recognition of the oral lesions. It must be emphasised, however, that simple visual recognition of the oral mucosal lesions may not be sufficient to provide a diagnosis in many instances. A variety of investigational techniques is applied to further study of these patients, most important being the biopsy. Oral mucosal biopsies are simple to perform and are often quite essential in obtaining a definitive diagnosis of many of the conditions illustrated in this atlas.

The terms commonly used in dermatology to describe lesions (for instance, macule, papule) may be used to describe oral lesions, However, because of the modified nature of the lesions in the oral mucous membranes, such terminology is much less widely applied. The modification of oral lesions which may make them difficult to recognise when compared to equivalent skin lesions depends largely on the nature of the oral environment. Frequently, the initial form of the lesion is made unrecognisable by the combined effect of repeated trauma, the continual presence of saliva and the invariable secondary infection which affects every oral lesion.

The final result of these factors is often the replacement of an easily identifiable primary lesion by a non-specific ulceration. This is particularly true of blistering lesions which may occur in the mouth – the detached or split epithelium is initially fragile and in the environment of the oral cavity the blisters rapidly break down to produce erosions and ulcers. (See figures **a, b, c.**) It is often necessary to await new and early lesions before coming to even a tentative diagnosis in some of these conditions.

a

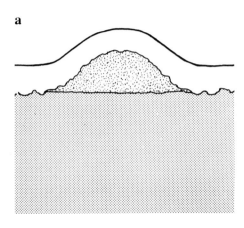

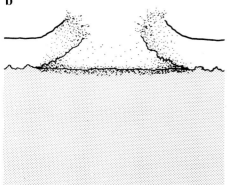
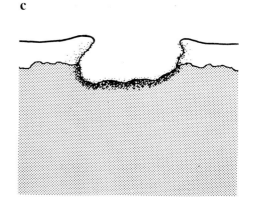

In this atlas an attempt has been made to illustrate the more common oral soft tissue lesions as well as rarities. A number of the conditions illustrated may appear in a wide range of clinical variants (lichen planus is a good example of this) and in these instances an attempt has been made to illustrate the complete range of variants. Histological sections have been introduced only when necessary to illustrate basic features reflecting on the clinical behaviour of the conditions described.

The order of the illustrations adopted depends entirely on clinical compatibility. Almost all more formal classifications suffer from disadvantages of one kind or another and there is no doubt that the present atlas could be classified quite differently. It is believed, however, that the present arrangement will be a convenient one and it is hoped that it will be of value not only to those working in the field of dentistry (and oral medicine in particular) but also to those working in other fields of medicine who may use the appearance of the oral mucous membrane as a diagnostic indicator.

Infections of the oral mucosa

The normal mouth contains a large number of organisms, many of them potentially pathogenic. In the patient with intact immune defences these organisms remain in a symbiotic relationship with the host. In patients with a reduced immune defence, however, certain of the organisms may act in a pathogenic manner. This is particularly true of *candida albicans*, an organism present in a high proportion of normal mouths, which produces lesions only when the host defence mechanisms are weakened. Oral candidiasis is therefore a sign of systemic abnormality and should be treated as such.

In other circumstances, however, lesions may be produced as a result of primary infection within the oral cavity. Primary syphilis and primary herpetic stomatitis are examples of this situation.

1 Primary herpetic stomatitis Primary herpetic stomatitis is the result of a first infection by the Herpes Hominis 1 virus and occurs most commonly in children and in young adults. The lesions are initially vesicular and may occur at any site in the oral cavity – usually they are widespread. The vesicles rapidly break down and it is unusual to see them intact. In this patient, however, the essentially vesicular nature of the lesions is still evident.

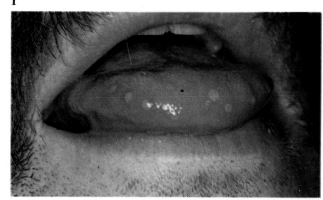

2 Primary herpetic stomatitis In this patient (aged six years) the vesicles have partially broken down with the production of ulcerated areas covered by yellow sloughs. Malaise, pyrexia and marked cervical lymphadenopathy are present. This is usually the case, particularly in children.

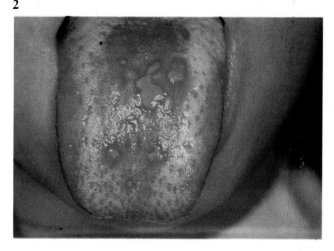

3 Primary herpetic stomatitis In primary herpes the majority of the lesions are confined to the oral mucosa although the lips and perioral skin may also be affected. The skin lesions are often more evidently vesicular, as in this patient.

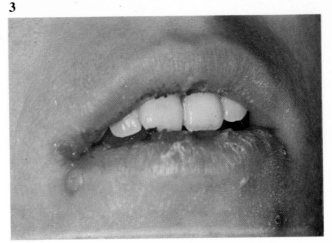

4 Primary herpetic stomatitis In this young patient the vesicles on the lips have broken down to form shallow erosions.

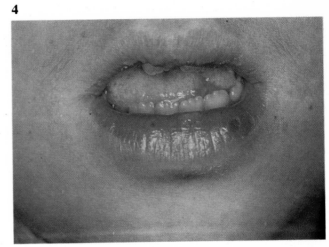

5 Primary herpetic stomatitis In the later stages of acute herpetic stomatitis, secondary infection plays an important part in the creation of discomfort and in the extension of the lesions. Stagnation occurs and the tongue may become heavily coated.

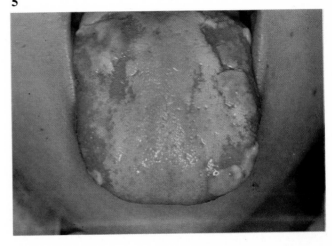

6 Primary herpetic stomatitis The breakdown and spread of the initial lesions is seen in this view of the commissure of a patient with widespread lesions of the mouth. A few small vesicles are still evident. At this stage the patient is often in considerable pain, largely due to the bacterial secondary infection. For this reason, the use of tetracycline mouth washes gives considerable relief although the viral infection is quite unaffected by this treatment.

6
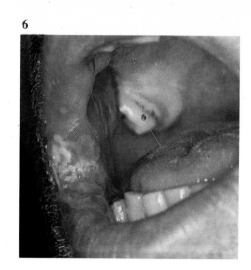

7 Primary herpetic stomatitis There may be a marked gingivitis, often associated with the retention of stagnation products. This leads to the appearance seen in this patient – a shiny, red marginal gingivitis contrasting with the white appearance of the rest of the attached gingivae. A developing gingival vesicle is also present.

7
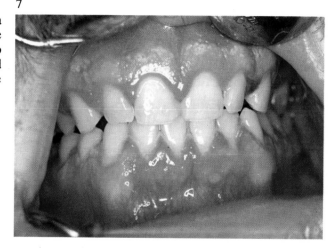

8 Primary herpetic stomatitis In the child patient the gingivitis is often marked and the swollen, red appearance of the papillae is not dissimilar to that seen in some cases of acute leukaemia. A blood examination is often necessary to differentiate between these possibilities.

8
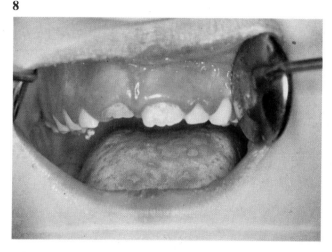

9 Recurrent facial herpes Following primary herpetic stomatitis the subsequent course of events depends largely on the integrity of the immune response of the patient. In approximately half of all patients the response is partially defective and persistently recurrent facial lesions may follow. These may be precipitated by trauma (such as excessive sunlight) or ill health (hence the popular name 'cold sore'). Even when widespread facial lesions occur it is very unusual for recurrent intraoral lesions to be found. In this patient erythematous pre-vesicular lesions are present, together with developing vesicles.

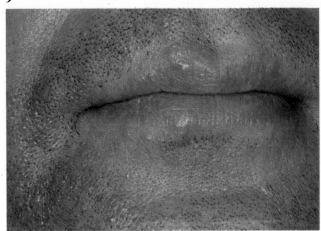

10 Recurrent facial herpes With the breakdown of the vesicles, crusted lesions are formed, in this case on the nose. Following healing (at 10–14 days from initial symptoms) viral material is thought to remain inactive within the tissues. Viral particles are not detectable in the skin during the quiescent phase and it is suggested that they may be present in the sensory nerves supplying the affected area. For this reason repeated recurrences often follow in the same area.

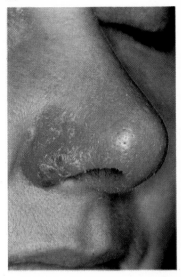

11 Herpes zoster Herpes zoster infections may occur on the face, closely limited to the cutaneous distribution of a sensory nerve. This is usually a branch of the trigeminal nerve but, in this case, C2 and C3 were involved. The lesions appear as a red papular rash which rapidly becomes vesicular, the vesicles often being haemorrhagic. Pain may be severe and there is often considerable malaise and fever.

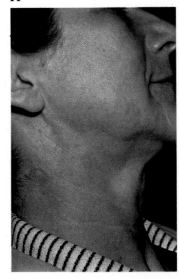

12 Herpangina This is caused by Coxsackie A4 virus and is a transient mild infection most often seen in children. Many small vesicles appear in the posterior part of the mouth and, in particular, on the soft palate. These are not particularly characteristic except, to some extent, by their posterior distribution.

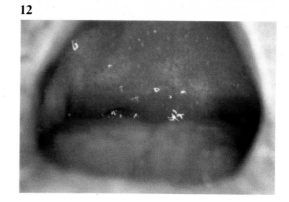

13 Hand-foot-mouth disease This disease is also caused by a Coxsackie virus (in this case, A16). As the name implies, this is an infection which produces lesions in the mouth (small ulcers) together with an erythematous vascular rash on the hands and feet. In the case illustrated only oral lesions were present – the diagnosis was made following viral antibody studies. This condition should be distinguished from the rare, and quite different, foot-and-mouth disease, caused by a virus normally carried by cattle.

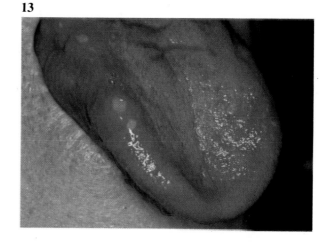

14 Acute pseudomembranous candidiasis (thrush) In this condition the candidal organisms are present on the surface of the mucous membrane as a network of hyphae in which are enmeshed epithelial cells, bacteria and debris, Some few hyphae penetrate superficially into the epithelium. If the pseudomembrane is wiped off, some epithelium is also removed and a bleeding surface is left; this may be considered a reasonable preliminary test in the differential diagnosis of thrush. This patient suffered from myasthenia gravis – a condition in which the immune response is weakened (see figure **65**).

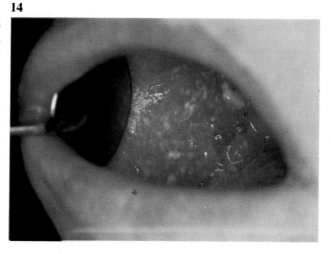

15, 16 Muco-cutaneous candidiasis This patient suffered from a deficiency of transfer factor with, therefore, a low resistance to candidal infection. The thrush-like lesions of the oral mucosa are associated with candidal infection of the finger-nails and toenails.

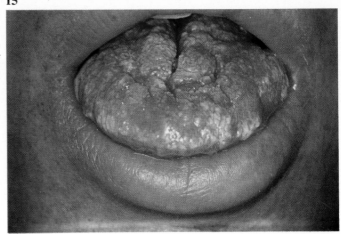

16 An infected finger-nail of the patient shown in figure **15**.

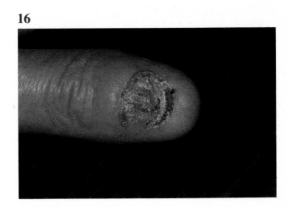

17, 18 Muco-cutaneous candidiasis A further patient with widespread oral lesions. The deep fissuring of the tongue is the end result of long-term chronic infection (see figure **65**).

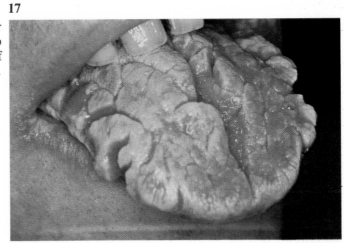

18 Muco-cutaneous candidiasis The candidal gingivitis is an unusual feature of the patient shown in figure **17**.

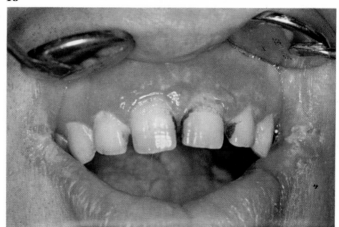

19 Acute atrophic candidiasis This condition resembles thrush without the presence of the superficial layer of hyphal organisms. The epithelium is atrophic and contains embedded hyphae. It readily breaks down to form painful erosions, as in this patient. The predisposing factor in this instance was an adrenal neoplasm (see figure **175**).

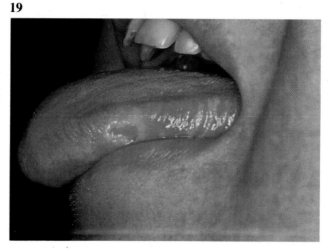

20 Chronic atrophic candidiasis This is an uncommon condition in the diffuse form illustrated. This patient, with a complex immune abnormality, shows atrophy of oral and vaginal epithelium with candidal infection.

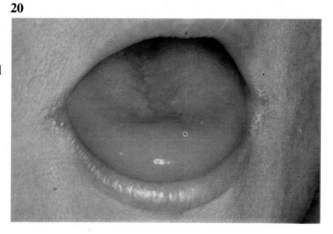

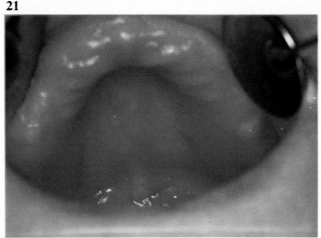

21 Chronic atrophic candidiasis (denture sore mouth) Denture sore mouth is a very common manifestation of candidiasis. It results from the secondary infection of traumatised tissues below a dental appliance – most often a full upper denture. The picture is of a painless erythema of the mucosa covered by the denture and restricted to it. Women are more often affected than men – the reason for this is not clear.

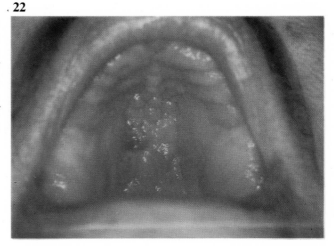

22 Papillary denture sore mouth In some cases the palatal mucosa below the full upper denture takes on a papillary appearance as in the present instance. There was evidence of candidiasis in this case and it is probable that this represents a hyperplastic response to trauma and infection. Another papillary hyperplasia of the palate with a different aetiology, is shown in figure **197**.

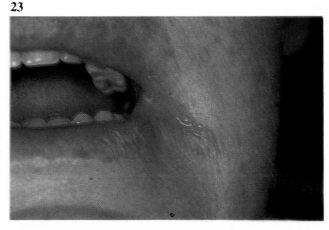

23 Candidal angular cheilitis This is commonly associated with denture sore mouth. It is encountered in patients with deep folds at the angles of the mouth, usually provoked or accentuated by the wearing of dentures of incorrect vertical dimensions. Ill health may also be a precipitating factor (see figures **136, 138**). The affected area is heavily infected by candidal organisms which thrive in the environment of moist warm skin. However, not all lesions of angular cheilitis are infected by candida – some are infected by bacteria (see figure **30**).

24 Granulomatous angular cheilitis In long standing cases of angular cheilitis, granulomatous areas may form – these are often highly resistant to treatment. In order to eliminate associated fissures it may be occasionally necessary to remove the granulations surgically.

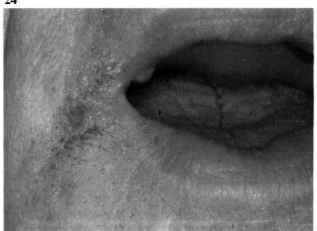

25 Primary syphilis (chancre) The primary syphilitic lesion appears as an indurated swelling some two or three weeks after infection. At first the surface is glazed but, as in this instance, the surface later becomes crusted. This case is unusual in that the long lasting primary lesion was in co-existence with lesions of the secondary stage – mucous patches and a skin rash (see figure **26**).

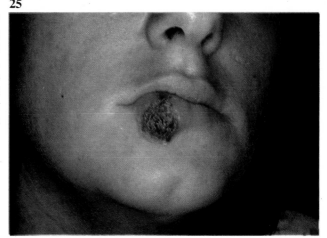

26 Secondary syphilis (mucous patch) Mucous patch of the buccal mucosa. Usually these are described as painless, but in this case the lesion was painful. These secondary lesions are heavily infected by *treponaema pallidium*, as are the primary lesions.

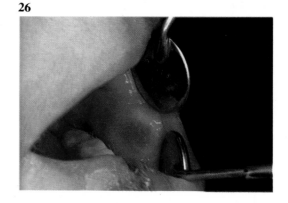

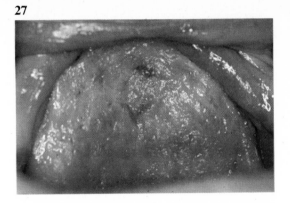

27 Tertiary syphilis (gumma) Gumma formation in the palatal mucosa has led to distortion of the tissues. Although not evident in the illustration, there was also marked loss of palatal bone in this patient, with the formation of a minute oronasal fistula.

28

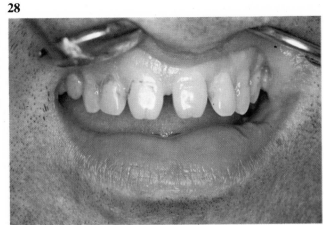

28, 29 Congenital syphilis In prenatal syphilis the spirochaetes may proliferate within the developing tooth germs with consequent distortion of tooth form. Shown here is a classical manifestation – Hutchinson's incisors (barrel-shaped and notched in the centre of the incisal edge).

29

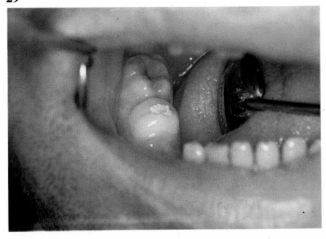

29 Moon's molars (rounded and with loss of normal anatomical detail) are a further classical manifestation of congenital syphilis.

30 Staphylococcal angular cheilitis A diffuse stomatitis due to staphylococci only is virtually unknown in the healthy patient. However, a high proportion of cases of angular cheilitis is infected by a staphylococcus, either alone or in conjunction with candida. It is impossible to differentiate between these on purely clinical grounds. In this patient the organism present was *staph. aureus*.

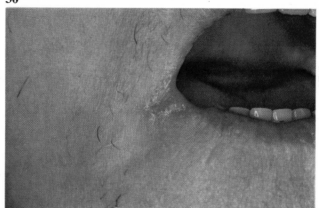

31 Staphylococcal pseudo-thrush In the heavily immunosuppressed patient the normal balance of flora is often grossly altered with a reduction in host resistance to infection. This may lead to infections by organisms which are usually thought to be commensal or to the onset of unusual lesions produced by pathogenic organisms. In this case, a staphylococcal thrush-like lesion had appeared on the tongue of a patient undergoing intensive immunosuppressive therapy for rejection of a renal transplant.

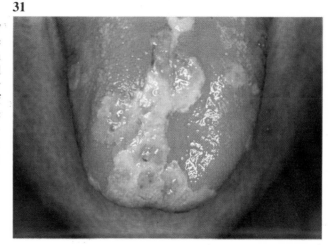

32 Tuberculosis Oral lesions of tuberculosis are now relatively uncommon but are almost always described as presenting in the form of an ulcer – usually secondary to pulmonary lesions. In this unusual case, the primary lesion was on the buccal mucosa, presenting as a faint white patch with erythematous areas and slightly indurated. Biopsy showed a tuberculoid structure and tubercle baccilli were incubated from the biopsy tissue.

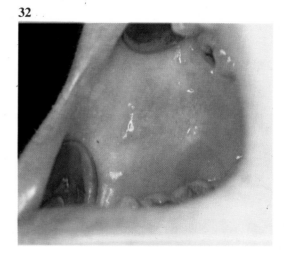

33 Tuberculous ulcer This lesion illustrates the more usual form of tuberculous ulcer, secondary to an active pulmonary lesion. However, with the great reduction in the number of cases of pulmonary tuberculosis, there has been a corresponding reduction in the incidence of tuberculous ulcers in the mouth and these lesions are now rarely seen.

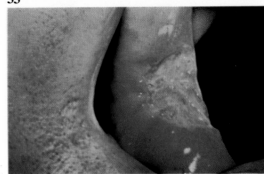

34, 35 Streptococcal stomatitis There is some controversy as to whether a true streptococcal stomatitis (or gingivitis) exists or whether this represents a misdiagnosis of a viral infection. However, there is no doubt that some few patients do present with a diffuse stomatitis in which the characteristics expected of a streptococcal infection are present and from which streptococci can be cultured. There is an associated tonsilitis and pharyngitis and systemic signs of mild toxaemia. The gingivae are red and shiny. The patient illustrated presented with all these features.

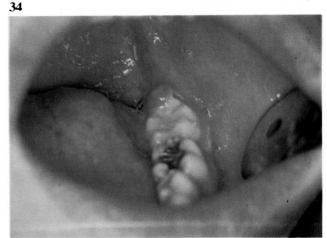

35 The gingivitis illustrated is characteristic of the condition described as streptococcal stomatitis (patient shown in figure **34**).

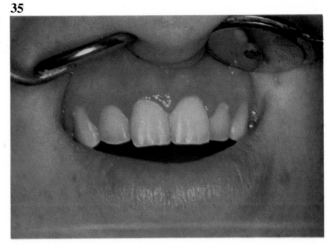

36 Acute ulcerative gingivitis The aetiology of this common gingival condition is not known, although there is always an associated overgrowth of Vincent's organisms (*Borrelia vincenti* and *fusiformis fusiformis*) in the affected areas. There is bleeding and tenderness of the gingivae with formation of shallow ulcers of the gingival margins and papillae. The typical destruction of the papillae is seen in this patient.

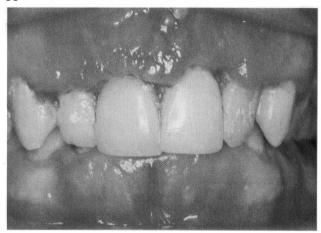

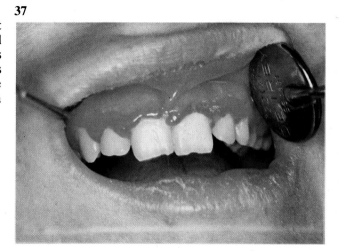

37 Acute ulcerative gingivitis In this patient an acute ulcerative gingivitis, with a marked overgrowth of Vincent's organisms, was secondary to an attack of acute herpes. This illustrates the opportunist nature of the proliferation of the organisms in the face of a weakened resistance.

38 Cancrum oris A combination of malnutrition, systemic disease and a viral infection provide the conditions for the rapid spread of infection by Vincent's organisms, which are responsible for the massive tissue destruction seen in cancrum oris. This condition is no longer encountered in European or North American conditions but still occurs in some African countries.

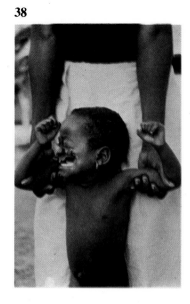

(See also figures **59–65, 143, 165, 166, 188, 189**.)

Recurrent oral ulceration

Recurrent oral ulceration is a common condition. Although there is a wide spectrum of clinical presentations most cases can be classified as one of the following three:
(a) Minor aphthous ulcers
(b) Major aphthous ulcers
(c) Herpetiform ulcers
There is not a clear understanding of the aetiology of any of these groups but it seems likely, on the present available evidence, that major and minor aphthous ulcers may represent a manifestation of auto-immune disease. Herpetiform ulcers are not due to infection by the herpes virus – the nomenclature is purely descriptive. Any of these three varieties of oral ulceration may be associated with genital ulceration or eye lesions. This condition is known as Behçet's syndrome and, in its fully developed state, destructive lesions are formed in the central nervous system, vascular system and joints. However, a restricted form of the syndrome with lesions of the oral and genital mucosae only is much more common. Recent work has shown a possible connection between oral ulceration and the existence of anaemias and latent anaemias of various types, and a clear association between oral ulceration and coeliac disease has also been demonstrated.

39 Minor aphthous ulcer This demonstrates the typical picture presented by a minor aphthous ulcer when present on a free surface. This is the most common form of recurrent oral ulceration and may occur at any age. Typically, one to five ulcers appear on the buccal or labial mucosa, floor-of-mouth or tongue. The palate and pharynx are virtually never involved in this form of ulceration. After being present for a variable period (usually about ten days), the ulcers heal without scar formation. There is a variable ulcer-free period before recurrence.

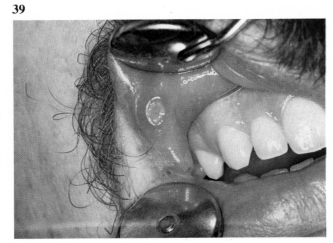

39

40 Minor aphthous ulcer When occurring in the depths of a sulcus, minor apthae present with a modified shape as elongated ulcers.

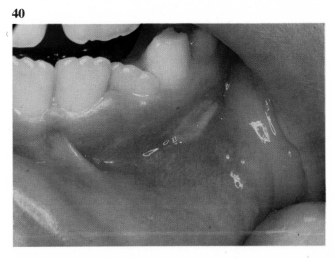

40

41, 42 Minor aphthous ulcer Aphthous ulcers may be precipitated by mild trauma as in the patient illustrated. The mild trauma from the fractured incisor, although not causing ulceration in itself, has stimulated aphthous ulcer production in the lower lip. Further mild irritation from the tooth has tended, in this case, to enlarge the size and prolong the duration of the ulcer. The ulceration in these cases is quite distinct from the simple traumatic ulcer (such as that seen in figure **43**) – it occurs only in those with a history of aphthous ulcers.

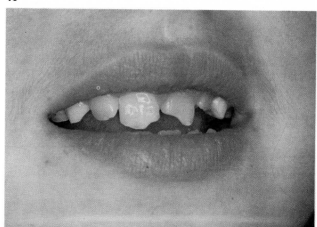

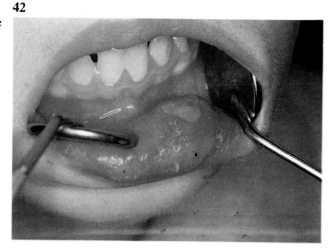

42 The ulcer precipitated by contact with the fractured incisor shown in figure **41**.

43 Traumatic ulcer This typical traumatic ulcer, with its punched out appearance and faintly white edge (caused by a minor change in the keratinization pattern of the epithelium), is included in this section to provide a comparison with the other ulcers shown. It was caused by the sharp edge of a fractured tooth.

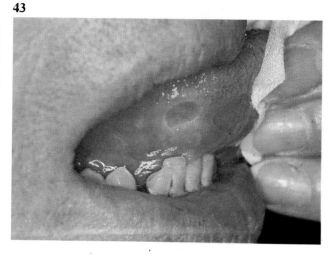

44   Major aphthous ulcer In general, major aphthous ulcers are larger than the minor variety and much longer lasting – up to several months in some instances. Characteristic of major aphthous ulceration is the involvement of the oropharynx and soft palate – as in the patient illustrated. On healing spontaneously these ulcers may leave severely scarred and distorted tissues (see figure **46**). If healing is accelerated by the use of systemic steroids, then scarring is much less marked (see figure **45**).

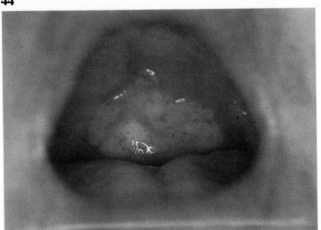

45   Healing major aphthous ulcer This is the ulcer shown in figure **44** in which healing has progressed rapidly under intensive systemic steroid treatment. Contrast this with figure **46**. In order to promote healing in this way, the dosages of systemic steroids required are high enough to cause adrenal suppression and many consequent side-effects.

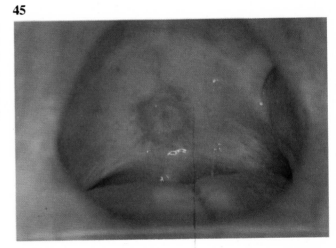

46   Scar formation in major aphthous ulceration In this patient repeated ulceration and scar formation in the soft palate has led to gross distortion. A further ulcer is present in the tonsillar area – a typical site.

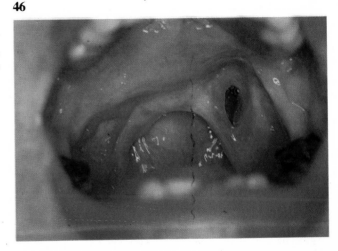

47 Herpetiform ulceration In this form of recurrent oral ulceration the ulcers are small and ill-defined but very painful. The site is characteristically at the front of the mouth – the lips, margins of the tongue and floor-of-mouth. There are usually many ulcers present in an attack – perhaps as many as fifty or one hundred. Occasionally a pre-ulcerative vesicular lesion may be seen. The duration of an attack is very variable and unpredictable. Most patients are female (2.6:1) and the 20–29 years age group is the most commonly affected.

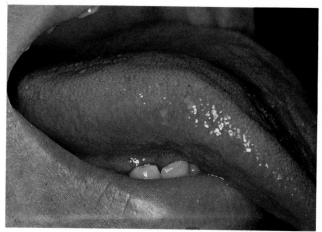

48 Herpetiform ulceration This patient shows all the characteristics of herpetiform ulceration. It is interesting that she was found to have coeliac disease and that treatment of this by controlled diet has led to a great reduction in the severity of her oral ulceration.

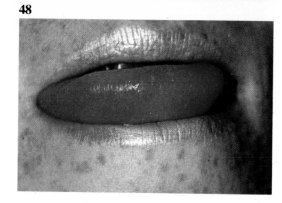

(See also figure **144**.)

The tongue and lips

Although many of the lesions illustrated in this atlas involve the tongue together with other areas of the oral mucosa, there are a number of conditions which specifically involve the tongue alone. These are largely dependent on the specialised nature of the tongue epithelium and, in particular, on the presence of the papillae which may undergo changes in their structure and distribution.

The lips do not have such a specialised structure. However, by being intermediate in site between the mucous membrane of the mouth and the skin of the face, some individual points of behaviour are reflected in the production of lesions confined to this area.

49 Microglossia Significant developmental abnormalities of the tongue are very rare, unless one includes minor variations in fissure patterns and size. Ankyloglossia (tongue-tie) is the most common and is associated, in this 13 year-old patient, with microglossia.

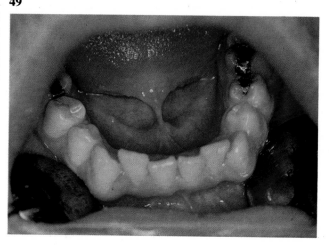

50 Microglossia This is the patient shown in figure **49** with the tongue fully extended. The restricted movement of the tongue caused by the tongue-tie is largely responsible for the lack of ability to protrude. While microglossia is almost invariably a developmental abnormality, macroglossia may occur in a variety of systemic conditions (see figure **179**).

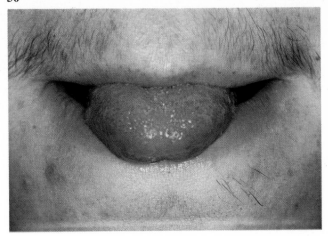

51, 52 Fissured tongue Deep fissuring of the tongue is quite normal in some patients. It may not be always evident, however, and these illustrations demonstrate how fissures may become either well marked or almost invisible according to the degree of lateral extension of the tongue. Although these deep, narrow fissures are of themselves symptomless, they may act as a site for infection and hence superficial irritation. This is due, presumably, to the anaerobic and static conditions they encourage.

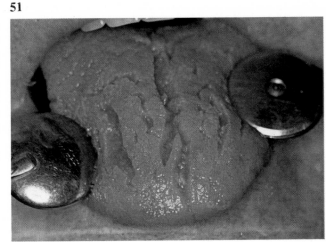

52 When laterally compressed, rather than extended, this tongue seems to display no unusual features.

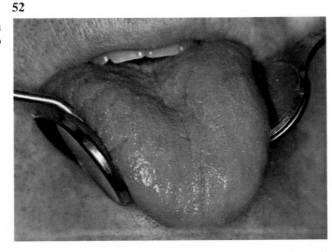

53, 54 Fissured tongue These illustrations demonstrate normal variations in tongue morphology. Figure **53** shows the form known as crenated tongue.

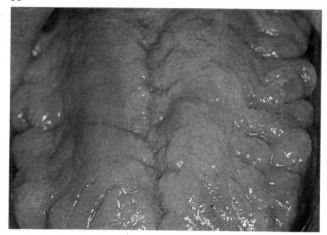

54 This shows the so-called scrotal tongue.

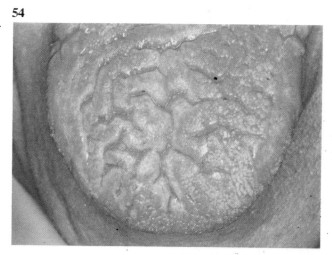

55 Melkersson-Rosenthal syndrome The three components of this syndrome are recurrent facial nerve palsy, facial swelling and a deeply fissured tongue. The aetiology is unknown and there is confusion in the literature between this condition, sarcoid and granulomatous cheilitis (figure **127**). It is reported that incomplete forms of the syndrome may occur, without abnormality of the tongue, but in this patient repeated bilateral episodes of facial palsy and swelling were associated with the deeply fissured tongue.

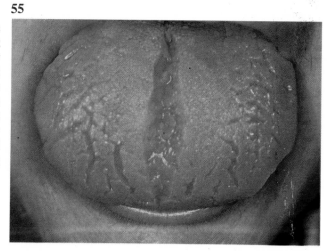

56, 57, 58 Hairy tongue This strange condition, brought about by elongation of the filiform papillae, is of unknown aetiology. Some cases (such as that shown in figure **58**) follow a course of antibiotic therapy but most are apparently completely idiopathic.

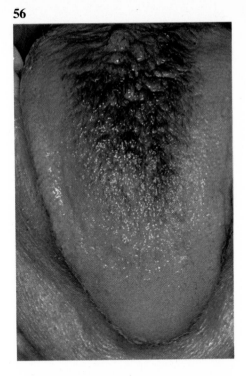

57 This demonstrates the susceptibility of fissured areas to pathological changes – in this case the enlarged papillae were restricted to the proximity of a deep midline fissure. The coloration (brown or black) is of unknown origin. It is usual to ascribe these colours to the presence of pigment-producing bacteria but, in fact, these cannot be demonstrated.

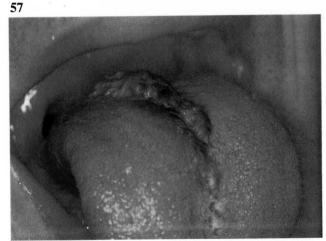

58 This black hairy tongue followed a course of systemic tetracycline, given for a respiratory infection.

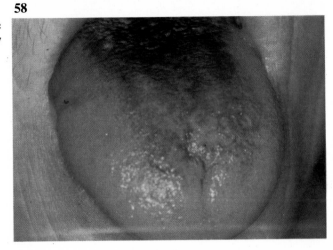

59, 60, 61, 62, 63, 64 Median glossitis The clinical presentation of median glossitis is very variable. That shown in figure **61** is of the so-called median rhomboid glossitis, long thought to be of developmental origin. It is now known that such a lesion represents a response to chronic infection by candida. This infection is poorly responsive to treatment and some authorities consider these lesions to be virtually irreversible. Occasionally (figure **62**), superficial ulceration may cause concern, the lesion bearing some resemblance to a carcinoma.

59

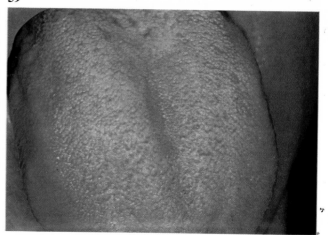

60

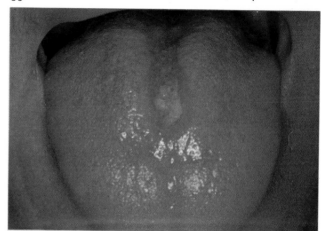

61

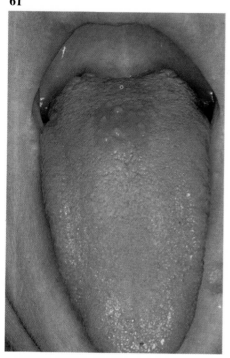

62

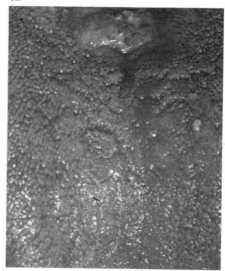

63 Median glossitis Very occasionally, there is a proliferative response to the infection, as in the patient shown here.

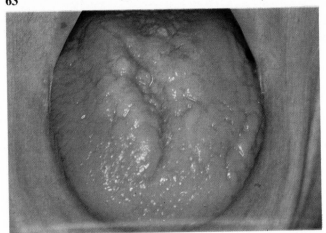

64 Median glossitis In this patient, the median glossitis appears as a red patch.

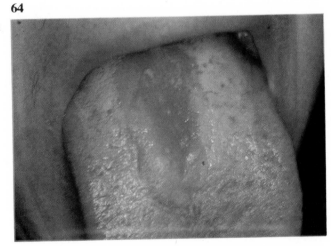

65 Pathologically fissured tongue In some cases of long standing infection scar production and pathological fissuring of the tongue may occur. In this instance the infection is candidiasis, the predisposing factor being myasthenia gravis. The infection had been present for many years (see figures **14, 18**).

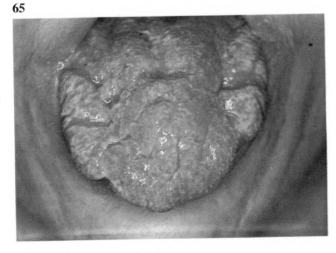

66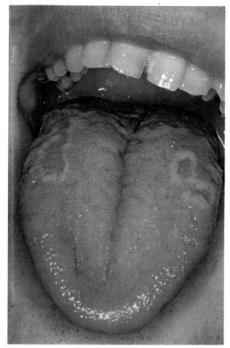

67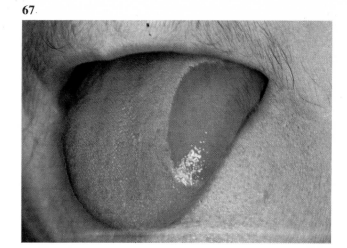

68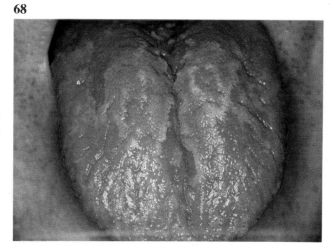

66, 67, 68, 69 Geographic tongue (erythema migrans) These illustrations show commonly occurring variants of the condition in which loss of the filiform papilla occurs temporarily. The name 'geographic tongue' well describes the map-like nature of the lesions, while the Latin term 'erythema migrans' indicates the apparent movement of the lesions over the surface of the tongue. This movement is due to the rapid appearance and disappearance of the lesions which start as small depapillated areas and then spread. The whole impression is that the lesions themselves are moving over the surface. A white margin to the lesions is almost invariable, although it may be quite faint. Figure **66** shows the typical condition although the other variants are not rare.

69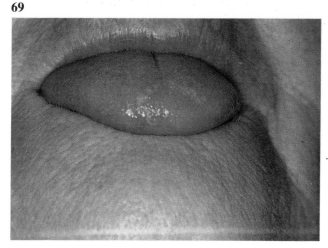

70 Depapillation of tongue Depapillation – the result of the loss of the filiform papillae – occurs in a variety of nutritional and haematological abnormalities. In this instance there was a multiple deficiency due to malabsorption. Serum iron, folate and B_{12} values were all reduced.

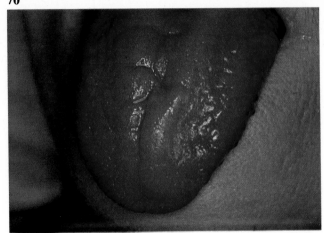

71 Lobulated tongue This example of a lobulated tongue in a severe folate deficiency-induced macrocytic anaemia, also shows the shiny surface associated with depapillation. Neither the depapillation nor the lobulation is associated with any specific generalised disease process.

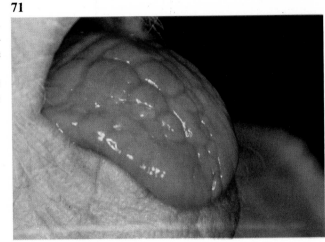

72 Sjögren's syndrome Mild fissuring of the tongue, giving a lobulated appearance, is seen in Sjögren's syndrome. This is not pathognomic, however, and similar patterns may be seen, for instance, in cases of haematological abnormality (see figure **71**). The components of the syndrome are salivary and lachrymal gland degeneration together with an auto-immune disease – often rheumatoid arthritis (see figures **235, 236, 237, 238**).

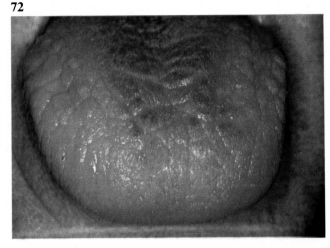

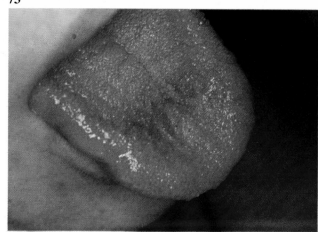

73 Antibiotic sore tongue (atrophic candidiasis) In some cases atrophy of the filiform papillae may follow a course of antibiotics. Secondary infection by candida may then occur and the tongue becomes red and sore. In this example, which followed a course of tetracycline therapy, there are areas of filiform atrophy, together with some rather brown 'hairy patches'.

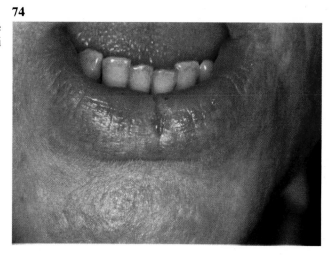

74 Median fissure of lip Fissures of this type are often secondarily infected by staphylococci and may be very persistent.

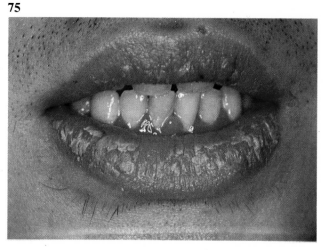

75 Exfoliative cheilitis This is a condition of unknown aetiology in which there is a grossly excessive production of keratin associated with increased mitotic activity in the basal layer. It is restricted to the vermilion border of the lips – predominantly the lower – and seems to be quite benign. A similar condition may be stimulated by the effect of sunlight (actinic cheilitis) but in the case of exfoliative cheilitis a precipitating factor cannot be found. It is very resistant to all forms of treatment.

76 Perioral dermatitis This condition, similar to rosacea, is confined to the perioral region and is seen most commonly in younger women. There is an overall erythema with the presence of small papules or pustules. The origin of this condition is not known but the use of powerful steroid ointments in the area is suggested as being one precipitating factor.

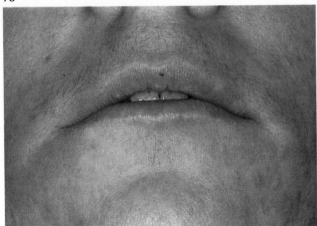

(See also figures **137–141, 202.**)

Oral lesions in diseases of the skin

As has been pointed out previously, there is a close relationship between the oral mucous membrane and the skin, and many essentially dermatological diseases result in the production of lesions of the oral mucosa. In some instances, the oral lesions may be the first to appear, by a considerable interval, and are thus of particular importance in diagnosis. From the point of view of treatment, also, the oral lesions may be of considerable significance in this group of disease since ulceration and secondary infection are common, leading to pain, discomfort and difficulty in eating.

LICHEN PLANUS

This is a disease of skin and mucous membranes which is relatively common and which is often seen in the oral medicine clinic. In patients reporting with skin lesions, some 70 per cent have oral lesions whereas among those reporting primarily with oral lesions, only 35 per cent are found to have skin lesions. This apparent paradox depends on the relative asymptomatic nature of many of the oral lesions and on the fact that the onset of the skin and mucosal lesions may be widely separated in time. When skin lesions alone are present the condition may be expected to last for a maximum of two years. When oral lesions are present, however, the condition is much longer lasting. The age range of patients is wide (30–80 years in most cases) with a preponderance of females (70 per cent). The oral lesions present with a wide range of appearances and the associated symptoms also vary greatly. All lesions, however, show the basic histological structure illustrated in figure **77**.

Approximately 30 per cent of patients with oral lichen planus present with the non-erosive form, the remainder having some degree of mucosal erosion.

77 The characteristic histological changes found in lichen planus of all types lie in the dermis. A dense band of inflammatory cells – mostly lymphocytes – lies below the epithelium which shows a wide range of reactions ranging from hyperkeratosis with acanthosis, to atrophy. The basal layer of the epithelium shows degenerative changes and the rete pegs are flattened (as here) or assume a saw-tooth configuration. Whatever the clinical variant of the condition, this basic histology is usually recognisable – both in mucous membranes and (with evident minor differences) in skin.

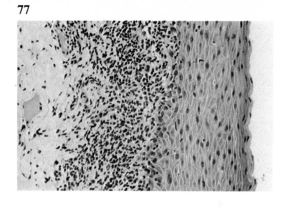

78, 79 Lichen planus – skin lesions The skin lesions of lichen planus appear as pink papules with white streaks on their surface (Wickham's striae). These may appear on any part of the body but mostly on the front surfaces of the wrists, genital skin, abdomen and lumbar regions. There may be itching – this is variable.

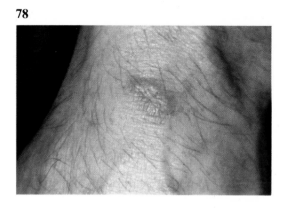

79 Scratching may precipitate the formation of lesions along the line of trauma – the Köbner effect.

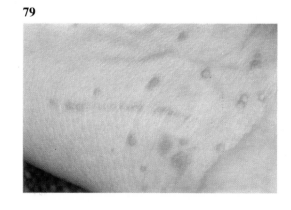

80 Lichen planus of inner canthus of eye Although this site is rare, the lesion is characteristic and shows fine Wickham's striae.

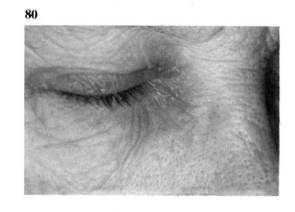

81 Lichen planus – alopecia If the scalp is involved – as it is occasionally – there may be patchy alopecia. This usually occurs in females and may be of cosmetic importance since scarring may result and the hair loss may become permanent.

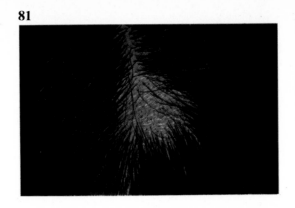

82 Reticular lichen planus This is the classical presentation, with white striae on the mucosa, arranged in a linear or reticular manner. These are thought to be the equivalent of the Wickham's striae of the skin lesions. The lesions cause little complaint and are often noticed incidentally. The buccal mucosa is affected in most cases of oral lichen planus of whatever type.

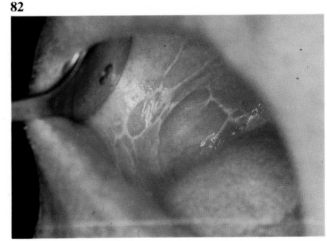

83 Reticular lichen planus A slightly modified reticular pattern as frequently seen on the tongue. Lesions of the tongue are present in approximately 27 per cent of all patients with oral lichen planus.

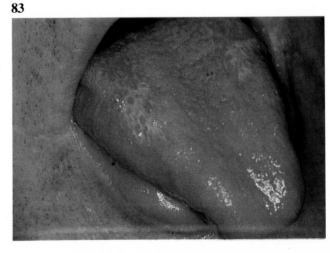

84 Confluent lesions of lichen planus The differentiation between such a lesion and a leukoplakia depends entirely on the histological appearances after biopsy.

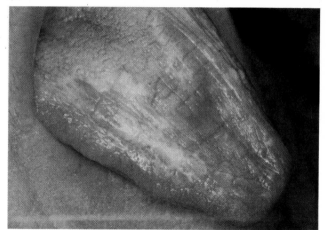

85 Confluent lesions of lichen planus In this lesion there is a hint of reticulation at the margins. The dense white area, although clinically suspect, presented the typical histological appearances of lichen planus.

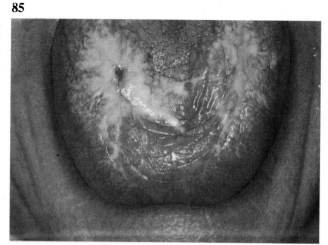

86 Minor erosive lichen planus The essential epithelial change in this form of the disease is of atrophy. There is practically always an associated area of non-atrophic lichen planus which gives a pointer towards clinical diagnosis. Approximately 65 per cent of oral lesions are of the minor erosive type.

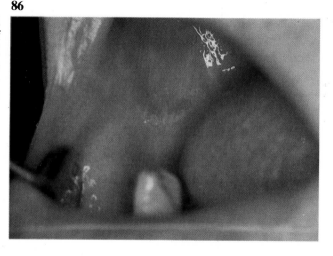

87   Minor erosive lichen planus In this case the lesions are more diffuse than that shown in figure **86**.

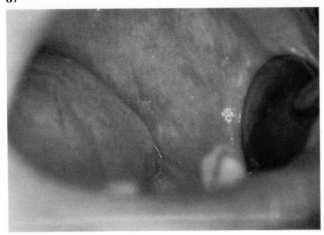

88   Minor erosive lichen planus of gingivae In this patient the gingivae are predominantly affected. The fragility of the gingival tissues in this situation led to the use of the largely superseded terminology of 'desquamative gingivitis'. The gingivae are affected to some extent in 25 per cent of cases of erosive lichen planus.

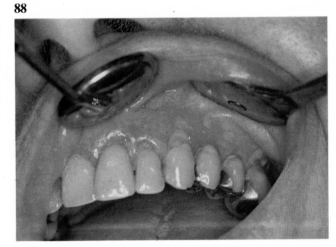

89   Minor erosive lichen planus of palate This is a relatively unusual site – affected in approximately 8 per cent of patients.

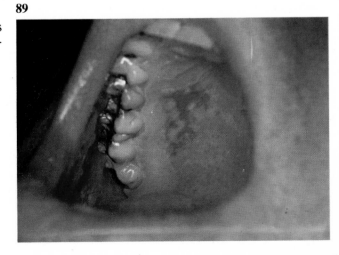

90 Lichen planus simulating leukoplakia This lesion closely resembles a leukoplakia of the commissure (see figure **184**). However, the histology was of lichen planus and, eventually the lesion regressed with others present in other parts of the mouth.

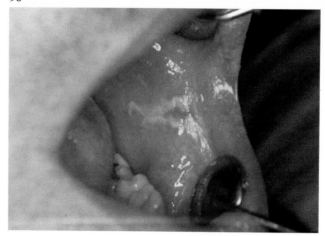

91 Lichen planus simulating erythroplakia This elevated red lesion was clinically diagnosed as erythroplakia (see figure **192**). Again the histology was of lichen planus and the lesion responded to therapy.

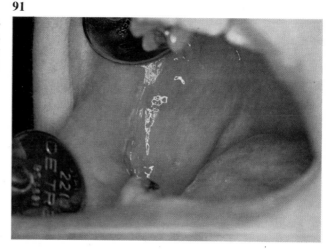

92, 93 Major erosive lichen planus In this relatively unusual variant (7 per cent of all cases) the lesions are remarkably different from those of the minor erosive form. This tends to occur in older patients, is of sudden onset and is usually widespread over the oral mucosa. The erosions present as clearly defined ulcers, covered by a raised yellow plaque with a glazed appearance.

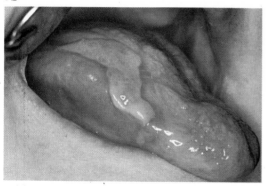

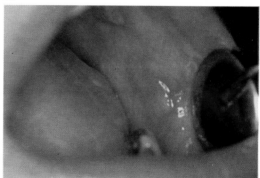

94 Major erosive lichen planus In some instances, virtually the whole of the tongue may be involved in the erosive process.

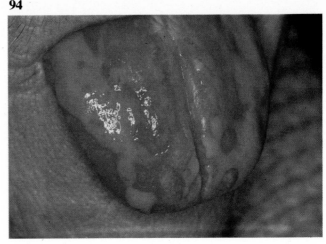

95, 96 Major erosive lichen planus – healing phase When healing, the major erosions of the tongue may regress leaving behind a white lesion (figure **95**). This, in its turn, eventually resolves leaving a smooth depapillated surface (figure **96**). This is the patient shown in figure **94**.

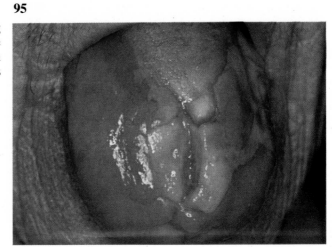

96 A further stage in the healing of the lesions shown in figures **94, 95**.

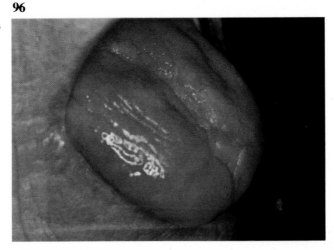

97 Major erosive lichen planus – non erosive areas Even when erosions are gross there is almost always some area of the non-erosive type present – often on the lower lip, as in this instance. This is the patient shown in figure **94**.

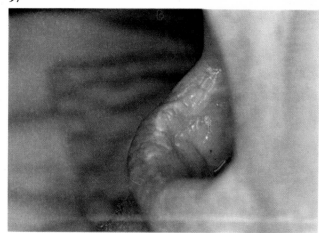

97

98 Bullous lichen planus With the degeneration of the basal layer of the epithelium the area is mechanically weakened and, rarely, the epithelium may lift to form bullae, as in this case. These bullae are short-lived and disintegrate to form characteristic erosions.

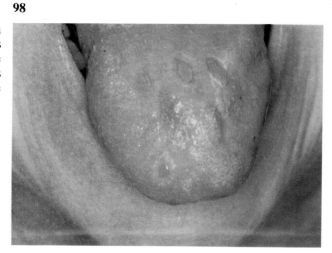

98

99 Lichen planus of lip with crusting In this patient, persistent trauma has modified the appearance of the lesion on the lower lip Spontaneous crusting of this kind does not occur in lichen planus but is a feature of some other conditions (such as chronic discoid lupus erythematosus) with which lichen planus might be confused (see figure **125**)

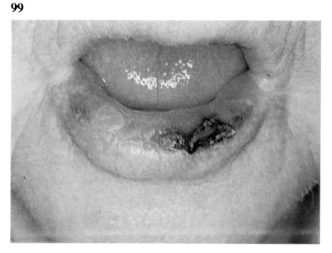

99

BULLOUS DISEASES

In this group of disorders, lesions present initially in the form of blisters caused by the collection of fluid below the epithelium or between its cells. Many patients have oral as well as skin lesions – in pemphigus in particular, the oral lesions may precede others by a considerable period. Diagnosis on the basis of the oral lesions is quite possible and may lead to the early institution of treatment. In this group of diseases both the skin bullae and those of the oral mucosa tend to rupture with mild trauma, leaving erosions as the most prominent features.

100   **Pemphigus – skin lesions** This lesion of the back of the hand clearly demonstrates the bullous nature of the disease process, although the blister fluid has already been lost. The next stage is the loss of the fragile epithelium to produce an erosion similar to those shown in figure **101**.

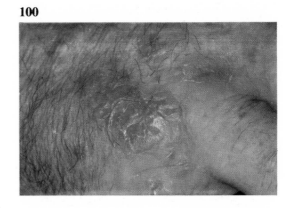

100

101   **Pemphigus – skin lesions** Multiple erosive lesions of the leg.

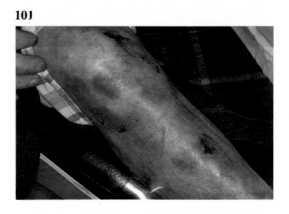

101

102   **Pemphigus – bulla of lip** In this instance the large bulla on the lip has been photographed at a very early stage. Within a short time this would be expected to disintegrate, leaving a mucosal erosion similar to those shown in figure **103**.

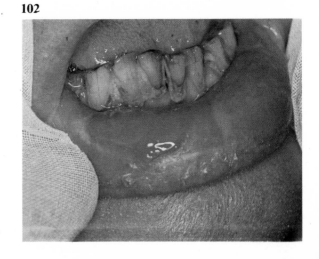

102

103 Pemphigus – buccal mucosa Widespread erosions have resulted from the rupture of multiple bullae.

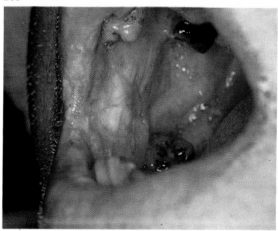

104 Pemphigus – early palatal lesions This is an early case of pemphigus in which oral bullae occurred before the onset of skin lesions. The rather fringed nature of the erosions caused by the splitting of the epithelium is characteristic.

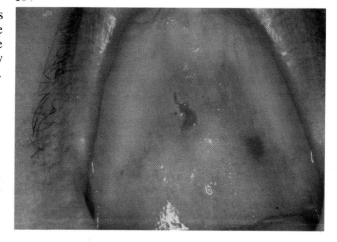

105 Pemphigus – histology In this section can be seen the intra-epithelial split which is the cause of the lesions. The floor of the bulla is lined by the remaining basal cell layer, while the fluid contains floating epithelial cells with the signs of acantholysis (loss of intercellular attachment) – these are known as Tzanck cells. Their presence is a valuable diagnostic feature if suitable bulla fluid can be obtained.

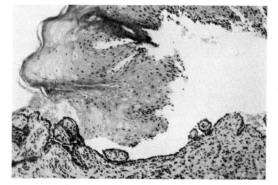

106 Pemphigus – antibodies In pemphigus, autoantibodies to intercellular substances and structures are found. In this section they are demonstrated by an immunofluorescent technique and can be seen around and between the cells. The exact role of these antibodies has not yet been determined.

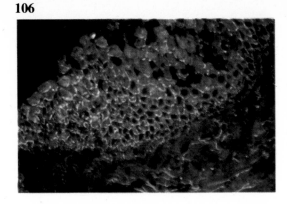

107 Pemphigoid – intact bulla of tongue In pemphigoid, the oral lesions tend to remain intact for a longer time than those of pemphigus and may remain evident, although ruptured (figure **108**)

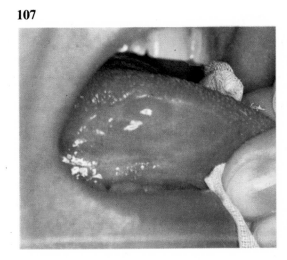

108 Pemphigoid – palatal lesion In this lesion a part of the ruptured bulla is still present in association with the eroded area.

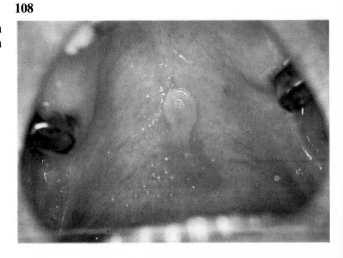

109 Pemphigoid – histology This section demonstrates the lifting of the intact epithelium from the underlying connective tissue. The bulla fluid contains no Tzanck cells.

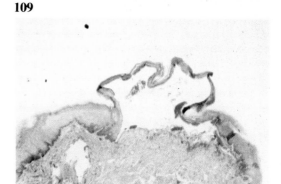

110 Pemphigoid – antibodies In pemphigoid, autoantibodies are found at the level of the basement membrane complex. Compare this to the intracellular antibodies demonstrated in pemphigus by the same technique (figure **106**)

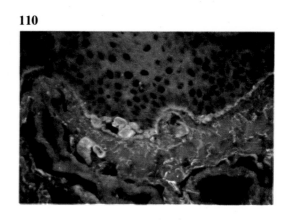

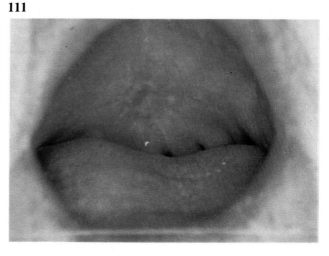

111 Benign mucous membrane pemphigoid In this condition the blisters are usually restricted to a relatively small area – in this case, the soft palate. The bullae, although usually relatively small, heal with scar formation. Since the eye is quite often involved adhesions may form in the conjunctival sac and the sight may be severely affected. This is usually a disease of old age.

112 Dermatitis herpetiformis There is some dispute as to what may be termed the 'typical' oral lesion in this blistering disease – erosions and bullae have been described. In this instance a lichen-like lesion appeared without, however, the histological appearances of lichen planus.

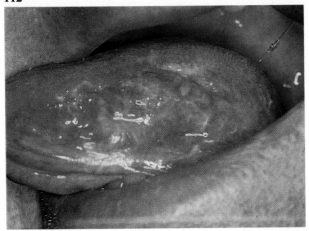

113 Epidermolysis bullosa – hand This genetically determined condition is one in which sub-epithelial blistering occurs and in which the dermal-epidermal junction is excessively fragile. The blisters and erosions heal with scarring; tissue distortion, with loss of nails, may occur. This is the hand of a severely affected six year-old girl.

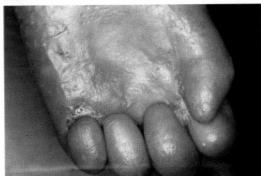

114 Epidermolysis bullosa – teeth and oral mucosa In this view of the patient shown in figure **113**, hypoplasia of the teeth is evident. Gross caries follows in such circumstances, since oral hygiene is almost impossible because of mucosal fragility. An erosion is visible on the gingivae. The scarring following the lesions may lead to restriction of opening or, as in this patient, binding down of the tongue.

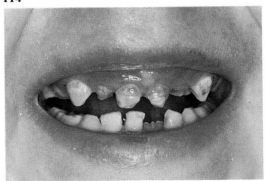

115 Epidermolysis bullosa – bulla formation The essentially bullous nature of the condition is shown by the multiple blisters in this patient (a boy of seven years, slightly less severely affected than the patient of figures **113** and **114**). Because of the fragility of the tissues, oral bullae are never seen in this condition.

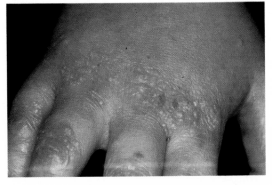

116, 117, 118 Erythema multiforme In each of these patients the characteristic crusting of the lips is evident. The rest of the oral mucosa may be involved as may the skin (figures **122, 123**) and other mucosae. The term 'Stevens-Johnson syndrome' is occasionally used to describe the more widespread form of this condition but there is no essential difference between this and the form restricted to the oral cavity. Even when the lesions are predominantly oral, the skin and other mucous membranes may be affected to a minor degree. Young adults are most commonly affected and the systemic effects may be quite severe, with fever and malaise. The aetiology of this condition is not known, but it is suggested that it may be an immune complex disease as a result of stimulation by a wide range of antigens.

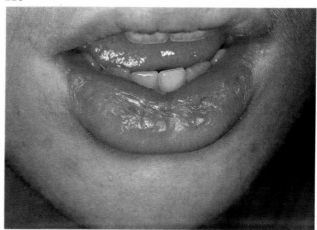

117 This is a further case of erythema multiforme in a young adult showing characteristic crusting of the lower lip.

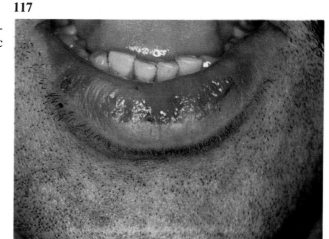

118 In this 16 year-old girl the involvement of the lower lip is unusually severe.

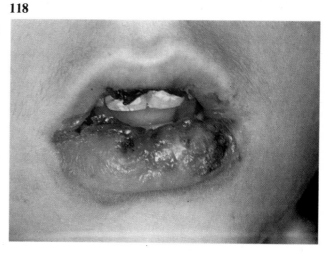

119 Erythema multiforme – palate In this instance the palatal mucosa is affected. Although, as is usual, the lesions have broken down to form erosions, the essentially bullous nature of the disease can be seen. Episodes may be precipitated by a wide range of factors – in this case by an attack of recurrent herpes – but in most instances an aetiological factor cannot be found.

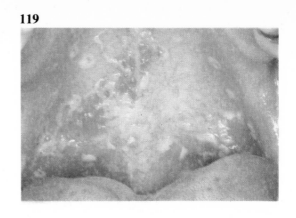

120 Erythema multiforme In this case, virtually the whole of the oral mucous membrane is affected. In cases such as this, clinical differential diagnosis from primary herpetic stomatitis may be difficult.

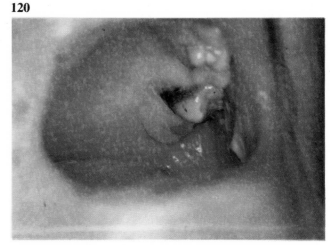

121 Erythema multiforme – restricted form The name 'multiforme' implies a range of morphology of the lesions and this, to some extent, extends to the clinical behaviour of the condition. In some few, usually older patients, the condition is less widespread and less severe in its effect. This patient is an example of this group.

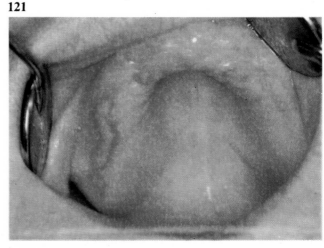

122, 123 Erythema multiforme – skin lesions
The characteristic skin lesions are iris ('target') lesions occurring predominantly on the hands, arms and feet. There may or may not be a central blister; if one is produced it is usually quickly lost with resulting scab formation (figure **123**). The condition of the patient shown in figure **122** was precipitated by the use of barbiturates and had recurred on a number of occasions. The presence of skin lesions settles the differential diagnosis between erythema multiforme and acute herpetic stomatitis – sometimes a difficult one if the oral mucosa alone is involved.

123 This shows a 'target' lesion with a central scab following rupture of a bulla.

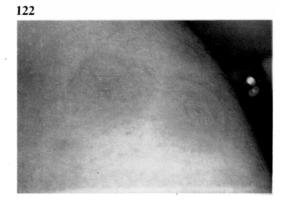

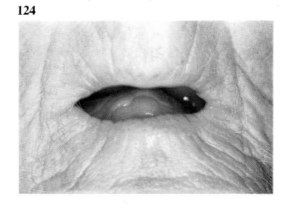

124 Generalised scleroderma Generalised scleroderma is a condition in which stiffness of the skin follows changes in the connective tissue. This may affect the mouth at an early stage, reducing the size of the oral aperture.

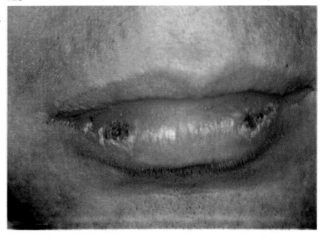

125 Chronic discoid lupus In chronic discoid lupus erythematosus a wide range of lesions of the oral mucosa has been described. The most usual lesion is of the lips, such as that illustrated. The combination of crusting and white keratinization is typical.

Lower gastrointestinal tract disease

Although there are indirect relationships between lower gut disease and abnormalities of the oral mucosa, there are relatively few situations in which comparable lesions occur in the two sites.

126 Crohn's disease – oral lesions Oral lesions occur in an appreciable proportion of patients with active gut disease. These take the form of granulomatous lesions as shown here on the buccal mucosa. The folding of the mucosa is characteristic and the hypertrophic tissue usually (but not always) has the characteristic histology of Crohn's disease. Painful oral ulcers may also occur, their severity fluctuating with that of the gut symptoms.

126

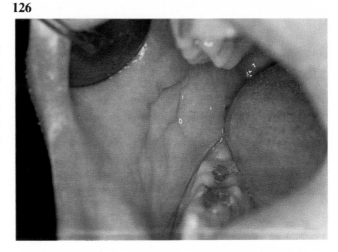

127

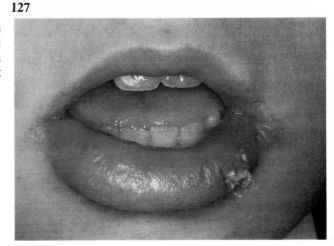

127, 128, 129 Chronic granulomatous cheilitis Closely associated with Crohn's disease, and probably a localised variant of it, this condition is marked by swelling of the lips – most commonly the lower lip.

128

128 In chronic granulomatous cheilitis there is angular cheilitis and a rather scaly condition of the perioral skin together with marked cervical lymphadenopathy.

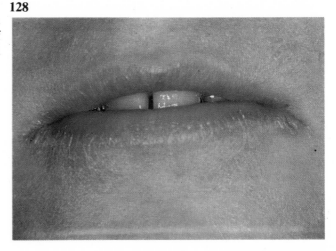

129 Intra-orally in chronic granulomatous cheilitis there are lesions closely resembling those of Crohn's disease and with their characteristic tuberculoid histological structure. This condition seems to affect adolescent patients and to become less marked in adulthood. It is not yet known whether Crohn's disease of the lower gut develops later in these patients.

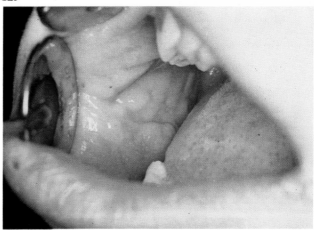

ULCERATIVE COLITIS

In ulcerative colitis about 5 per cent of patients have skin lesions. These include pyoderma vegitans, a non-specific pustular eruption, and pyoderma gangrenosum – a much more destructive condition in which burrowing pustules are formed which then break down to produce large ulcers. The lesions illustrated are thought to be equivalent to these skin lesions and are tentatively described as pyostomatitis vegitans and pyostomatitis gangrenosum, respectively.

130 Pyostomatitis vegitans – lower lip

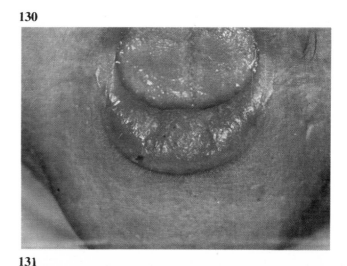

131, 132, 133 Pyostomatitis gangrenosum These destructive lesions of the oral mucosa were present in a patient with a non-specific ulceration of the colon – not diagnosed as classical ulcerative colitis.

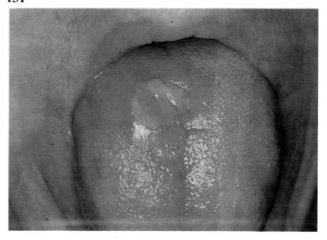

132 Pyostomatitis gangrenosum This illustrates a lesion of the lower lip in the patient shown in figure **131**.

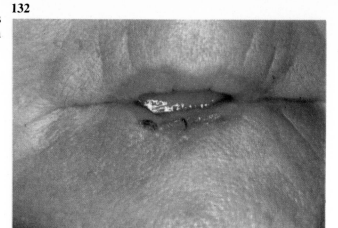

133 Pyostomatitis gangrenosum Healing of the lesion shown in figure **132** was associated with marked deformity.

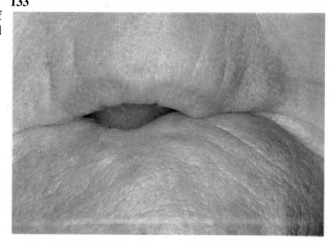

134, 135 Peutz-Jegher's syndrome This condition is transmitted as an autosomal dominant characteristic. The two features of the syndrome are the presence of intestinal polyps and a circumoral distribution of melanotic macules. The polyps are regarded as benign adenomas, but there are cases of malignant transformation recorded. The case illustrated is of a 13 year-old girl for whom a partial gut resection has been carried out. The patient's father has a similar history.

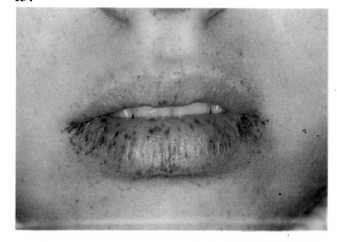

135 In the Peutz-Jegher's syndrome there is a secondary distribution of melanotic macules across the bridge of the nose.

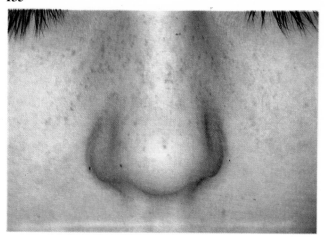

Disorders of blood and nutrition

Oral signs and symptoms may appear in a wide range of disorders of the blood – those affecting the erythrocytes and iron transport mechanism, those affecting the leukocytes and those affecting the platelets.

Patients with anaemias, latent anaemias and associated conditions may present with a wide range of oral manifestations, the result of metabolic changes in the oral mucosa. The oral changes are largely non-specific and may occur in the early stages of the blood disorder – often before the onset of changes in the morphology of the erythrocytes. The tongue is often affected by the atrophy of the papillae, the surface then appearing red and smooth. Apart from obvious changes, patients may complain of loss of taste sensation, or of generalised oral soreness. The changes in anaemias are closely linked with abnormalities in the nutritional factors which affect erythrocyte production – in particular vitamin B_{12} and folic acid. It should be remembered that the basic aetiology in many haematological disturbances is an abnormality of nutrition or the gastrointestinal tract.

In leukaemias and similar conditions, lesions may arise either as a result of the primary disturbance of metabolism of the tissues, from the deposition of malignant cells in small tumour-like aggregations in the mucosa or, occasionally, as a result of the cytotoxic treatments involved.

136

136 Iron deficiency This 16 year-old girl was found to have a haemoglobin of 5g/100ml. Her main complaint was of angular cheilitis and generalised oral tenderness. In this case the iron deficiency was consequent to excessive menstrual loss.

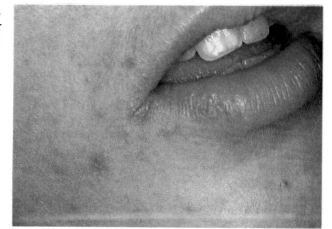

137 Latent iron deficiency This patchy depapillated tongue occurred in a patient with a much reduced serum iron concentration. The haemoglobin was not markedly reduced.

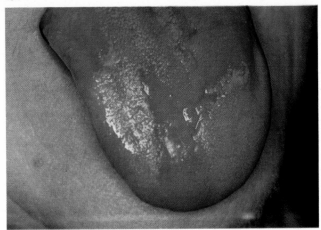

138, 139, 140 Folic acid deficiency In folic acid deficiency the most marked oral manifestation is often a glossitis. The tongue becomes red and painful and the papillae atrophy, leaving a shiny smooth surface. The serum folate levels in the patients illustrated were 1.7 µg/1 (figure **138**) and < 1 µg/1 (figure **139, 140**) – normal values being 3–20 µg/1.

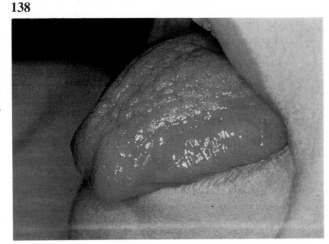

139 In folate deficiency angular cheilitis may be marked.

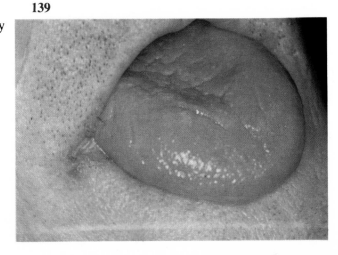

140 In this patient painful oral ulcers were associated with folate deficiency.

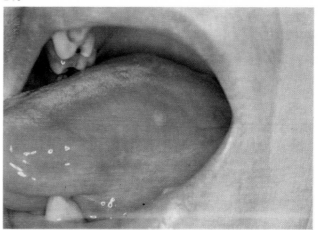

141 Vitamin B$_{12}$ deficiency B$_{12}$ deficiency may show itself initially by the presence of a sore tongue – as in this case. The red sore tongue, with atrophy of the papillae is often present in pernicious anaemia and, in the case illustrated, angular cheilitis is also present. This must be regarded as relatively uncommon since it has been reported only rarely. Although the case illustrated is of pernicious anaemia it should be remembered that B$_{12}$ deficiency may have other aetiologies (see figures **142, 143, 144**).

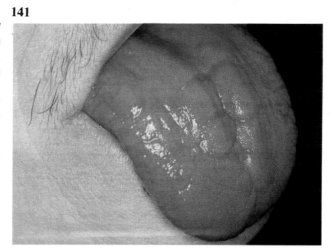

142 B$_{12}$-Folate deficiency This patient illustrated suffered from a complex malabsorption syndrome resulting in much lowered serum folate and B$_{12}$ levels. The peripheral blood film showed a macrocytic anaemia and the marrow was megaloblastic. There was a generalised stomatitis, ulceration and gingivitis.

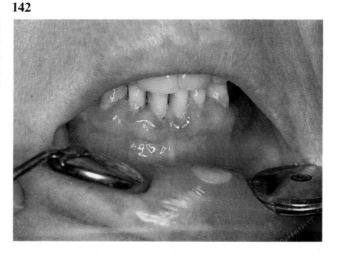

143 **B_{12}-Folate-Iron deficiency** The patient illustrated had undergone gastrectomy for a carcinoma of the stomach some fifteen years previously. There were marked deficiencies in the circulating levels of B_{12}, folate and iron and an intractable candidiasis was present on the tongue. Restoration of nutritional factors and antifungal treatment eliminated the pseudomembranous candidiasis, but below the affected areas were patches of candidal leukoplakia which necessitated cryosurgical treatment.

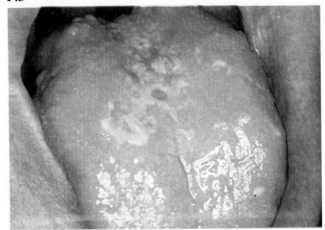

144 **B_{12}-Folate deficiency** In this patient, with a relatively minor problem of malabsorption, the serum B_{12} and folate levels were moderately depressed. The oral lesions present were similar in appearance and behaviour to minor aphthous ulcers but ceased to occur following treatment of the malabsorption and restoration of the normal circulating levels of the depressed factors.

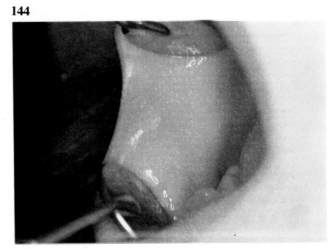

145, 146 **Acute myeloid leukaemia** A marked gingivitis, often with bleeding, may be an early sign of acute leukaemia.

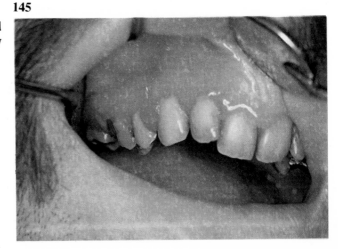

146 In this relatively advanced case of acute myeloid leukaemia there is a large palatal ulcer and hypertrophic changes in the palatal gingivae.

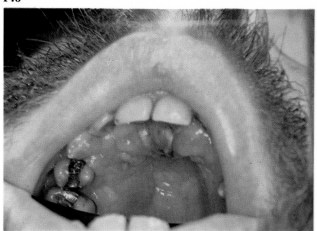

146

147, 148 Acute myeloid leukaemia In this patient small lymphoma-like deposits have been laid down subcutaneously.

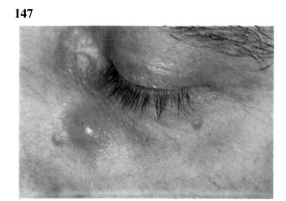

147

148 The lymphoma-like deposits present in the oral mucosa have broken down to form painful and persistent ulcers.

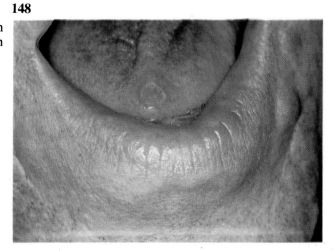

148

149 Agranulocytosis In agranulocytosis the lack of the protective granulocytes leads to widespread infective episodes, expressed in the oral cavity as severe ulceration. Apart from the mucosal ulceration this young male patient had undergone repeated episodes of respiratory tract infection.

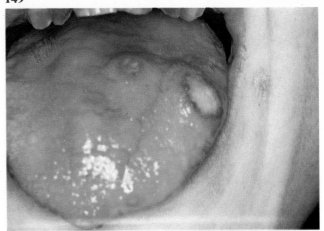

150 Thrombocytopenia A reduction in the number of circulating platelets may be shown up early in the oral cavity by the appearance of petechial haemorrhages, in this case on the soft palate. It should be remembered, however, that similar but transient petechiae may occur during the course of a common cold.

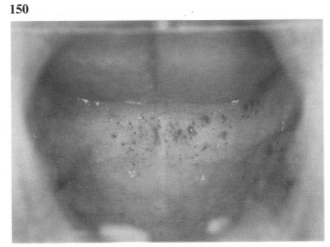

151 Vitamin C deficiency (scurvy) The characteristic oral change in scurvy is a gingivitis, the papillae being swollen, with a purple tint and are fragile. The patient with scurvy often has a grossly neglected oral hygiene and this (as in the patient illustrated) may cause further gingival inflammation.

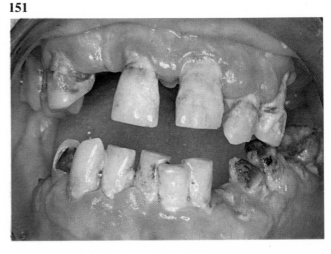

(See also figures **48, 202**.)

VASCULAR ABNORMALITIES

152, 153 Sublingual varicosities Enlarged veins on the undersurface of the tongue are frequently seen in older patients and may be considered a normal finding.

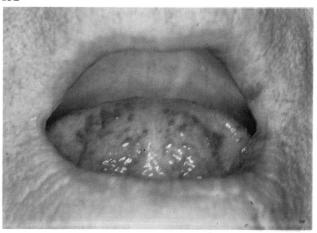

153 In an exaggerated form, marked sublingual varicosities may be a sign of hypertension and peripheral vessel incompetence.

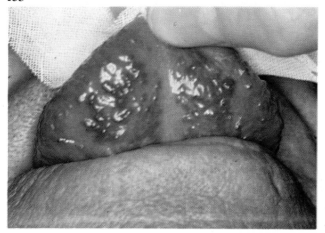

154 Haemangioma Haemangiomas have been variously regarded as benign neoplasms or as hamartomas. The usual criteria of growth of neoplastic lesions are difficult to apply since changes in haemodynamics are known to affect the size of haemanigiomas. The lesion illustrated had remained quite static over many years. (see figure **216**).

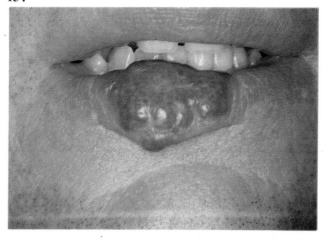

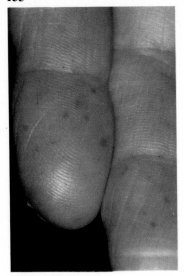

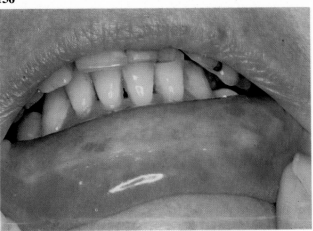

155, 156 Hereditary haemorrhagic telangiectasia (Rendu-Osler-Weber disease) In this genetically-determined condition small areas of dilated blood vessels appear on the skin and mucous membranes. The skin lesions may appear anywhere on the body and the oral mucous membranes are almost always involved. In more severely affected patients spontaneous haemorrhages may occur – most commonly in the form of epistaxis.

157, 158 Wegener's granulomatosis (thigh and gingivae) This condition is included in the present section since the basic aetiology is thought to be a vasculitis although the reason for this is unclear. Some other lesions (for example, pyostomatitis gangrenosum, figure **131**) probably have a similar aetiology but are classified differently for reasons of clinical convenience. In Wegener's granulomatosis the predominant lesion is a destructive granuloma which may occur in a number of sites – particularly in the respiratory tract, kidney and skin. These lesions may occur also in and about the oral cavity. A further oral abnormality in this disease is the presence of a peculiarly granulomatous gingivitis (figure **158**) which may occur early in the disease process and in the absence of destructive oral lesions.

158

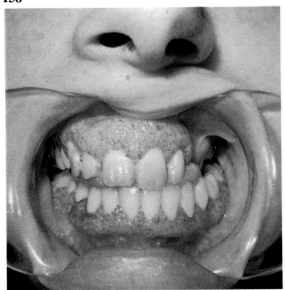

157

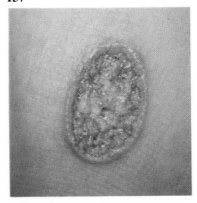

Drug-induced changes in the oral mucosa (including chemical burns)

159 Chemical burn of tongue (sodium hydroxide) This demonstrates a relatively mild degree of chemical burn of the tongue, the damage being largely due to depapillation. The lesion was caused by the incautious use of a pipette with a dilute solution of sodium hydroxide. Contact was transient.

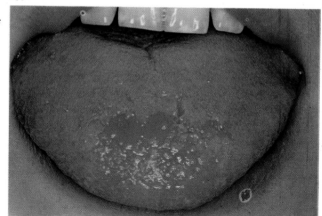

160 Chemical burn of tongue (root treatment medicaments) This more severe burn was caused by the leakage of a root canal sterilizing agent which was held in contact with the tongue for some time. Healing was slow – over a period of some two weeks.

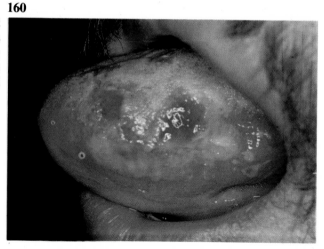

161 Aspirin burn The leukoplakia-like lesion characteristic of aspirin burn is usually seen in the buccal sulcus, close to a carious tooth. Such a lesion can be produced by the dissolving of a single aspirin-containing tablet in the area.

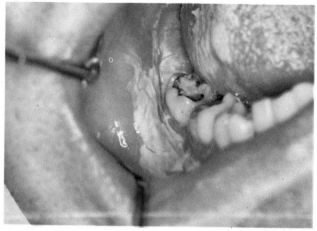

162, 163 Allergic reaction to penicillin (hand and tongue) The characteristic skin rash of the patient allergic to ampicillin is well known and is shown here.

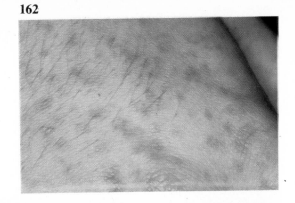

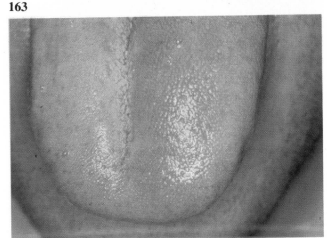

163 No more than a very small proportion of patients reacting to penicillin show oral symptoms. In the patient illustrated the oral reaction took the form of an angioneurotic oedema of the tongue, occurring unilaterally.

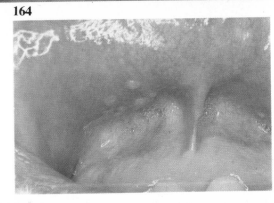

164 Allergic reaction to tetracycline The most common reaction to the use of oral topical tetracycline therapy is the appearance of the so-called antibiotic sore tongue (see figure **58**), not an allergic phenomenon. The patient illustrated here exhibited a vesicular reaction of the labial mucosa together with some mild and transient skin irritation – probably a true allergic reaction.

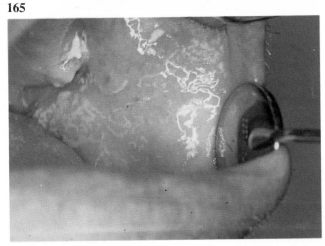

165 Steroid-induced candidiasis The role of systemic corticosteroids in the precipitation of oral infections has been illustrated in figure **31** by a staphylococcal lesion. However, oral candidiasis is a much more commonly induced condition, as in the patient illustrated. Acute pseudomembranous candidiasis (thrush) may be induced, not only by the use of relatively large dosages of systemic steroids as in this instance, but also by the use of local steroid applications in relatively low dosages.

166 Steroid-induced atrophic candidiasis In some patients on long term steroid therapy the oral mucosa becomes thin and atrophic. This may occur below denture fitting surfaces where the lesion appears as a particularly intractable 'denture sore mouth'.

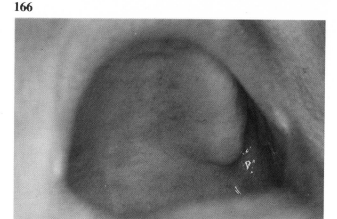

167 Gingivitis associated with cromoglycate and steroid aerosols Occasional patients under treatment for asthma with inhalations of sodium cromoglycate present with a spongy gingivitis involving predominantly the upper anterior gingivae. The aetiology of this is not clear – the patients seen with this condition also used occasional steroid inhalations and it may well be that these are an important factor. The condition appears to fluctuate in intensity over a period of time.

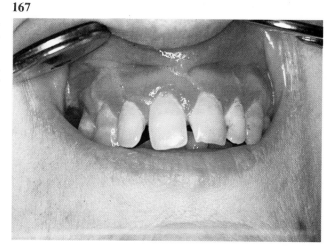

168 Azathioprine reaction Many of the potent cytotoxic and immunosuppressive drugs used in the treatment of malignancy or severe auto-immune disease may cause oral lesions. In this instance the use of azathioprine for the treatment of severe oro-genital ulceration produced a patchy depapillation of the tongue, not dissimilar in appearance to geographic tongue. The depapillation was reversed on the withdrawal of the azathioprine.

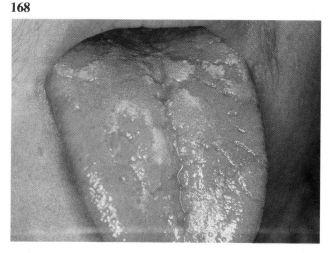

169 Phenytoin (epanutin) hyperplasia Hyperplastic gingivitis consequent to the treatment of epilepsy by phenytoin is a well-established complication. The characteristic appearance is of individual enlargement of the interdental papillae, the surface being stippled. In the later stages and if treatment is not given, secondary inflammatory changes supervene, and the texture of the hyperplastic gingivae becomes less firm. The aetiology of the gingivitis is not known; it is suggested that it may represent a hypersensitivity reaction but there is no clear evidence for this. Careful oral hygiene is said to eliminate the condition completely and there is no doubt that there is a relationship between lack of hygiene and the degree of hyperplasia.

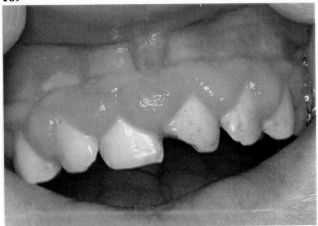

169

(See also figures **58, 73**.)

Endocrine disturbances

170 Diabetes mellitus There is some difference of opinion as to the degree to which the oral tissues are affected in diabetes mellitus. In some instances, oral infections (including candidiasis) may be an early sign of uncontrolled diabetes but these are by no means specific. It is generally accepted, however, that patients with diabetes mellitus have an exaggerated tendency towards periodontal disease. In general, and particularly in the stabilised patient, this periodontitis is not gross and the patient illustrated here shows a somewhat greater change than might be expected. Many other factors, such as the degree of plaque control, must enter into the aetiology. It has recently been suggested that there is a connection (via a common HLA linkage) between maturity onset diabetes and lichen planus. The patient shown in figure **84** has such an association.

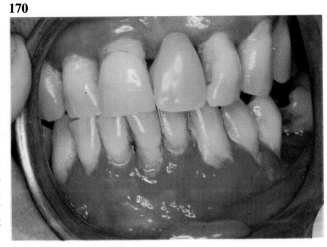

170

171 Pregnancy gingivitis There is a wide range of opinion regarding pregnancy gingivitis and its aetiology. It is generally accepted, however, that during pregnancy hormonal changes occur which make the gingivae unusually susceptible to inflammatory change. As in phenytoin-induced gingival hyperplasia, it is undoubtedly the case that strict oral hygiene will greatly reduce, or eliminate, the symptoms. The characteristic changes, apparently occurring in individual papillae, are seen in this relatively mild case.

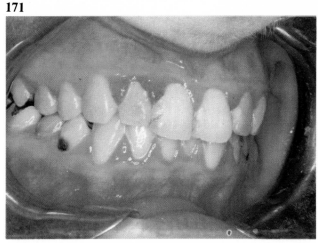

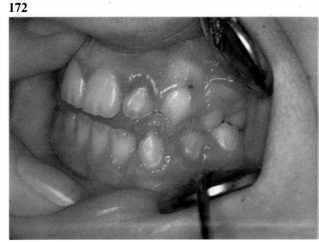

172 Puberty gingivitis A similar situation to that of pregnancy gingivitis may occur at puberty, particularly in females. Changes in hormonal balance lead to increased susceptibility of the gingivae to irritation and hyperplastic gingivitis is the result. Just as in pregnancy gingivitis, it is considered that stringent oral hygiene measures will eliminate the symptoms.

173, 174 Hypoadrenocorticalism (Addison's disease) In this patient, autoimmune destruction of the adrenal cortex has occurred and is associated with chronic mucocutaneous candidiasis. Unlike the patient shown in figures **15, 16** in which the mucocutaneous candidiasis has a different aetiology, the oral mucosal changes are of atrophic candidiasis rather than that of pseudomembranous candidiasis. The finger-nails are similarly affected, however. In most cases of Addison's disease the earliest evident oral change is of pigmentation of the mucosa (as in the patient shown in figure **176**).

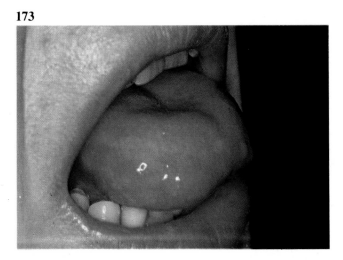

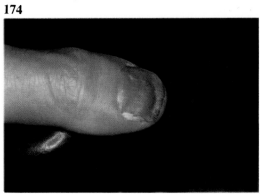

175 Hyperadrenocorticalism (Cushing's syndrome) In this patient there is widespread oral candidiasis, both pseudomembranous and atrophic (see figure **19**). The primary aetiological factor in this case is an adrenal tumour causing a gross overproduction of natural corticosteroids. Just as in the case of therapeutic treatment with large doses of corticosteroids, the immune response to candida is suppressed.

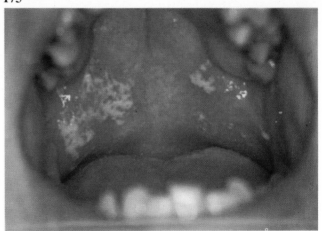

176 Melanotic pigmentation – Addison's disease In hypoadrenalism melanotic spots may appear on the skin and on the oral mucosa, in almost any site. In this patient the pigmentation was confined to the palate. Examples of pigmentation of the oral mucosa of non-endocrine origin are shown for comparison in figures **177, 178**.

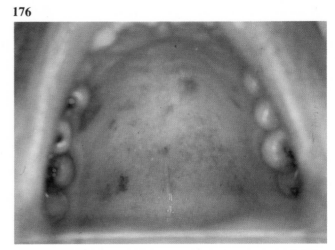

177 Melanotic pigmentation – racial The distribution of racial melanotic pigmentation in the oral cavity is widely variable. In this patient the patchy nature of the pigmentation, together with a slight superimposed smoker's irritation of the minor palatal glands, produces a bizarre effect.

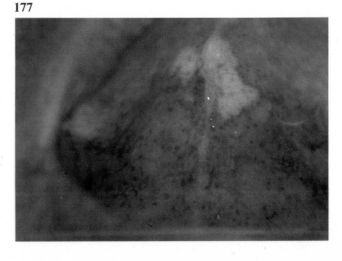

178 Amalgam pigmentation The traumatic implantation of amalgam is by far the most common cause of black patches on the oral mucosa. However, after some time has passed (during which the metal becomes distributed and so invisible on x-ray) the differential diagnosis from a melanoma may be difficult. This is such a case – the site is most unusual.

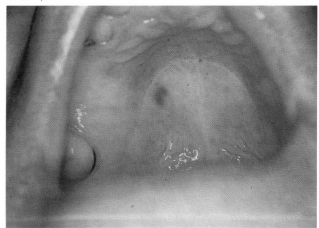

179, 180 Acromegaly In acromegaly two types of oral manifestation are seen – enlargement of the tongue and lips, and bone growth. The enlarged tongue overlying the occlusal surfaces of the posterior teeth is illustrated.

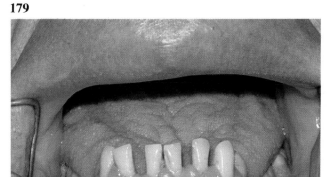

180 Bone growth in the maxilla in acromegaly is shown by the comparison of the position of the natural teeth with that on the partial denture, made some two years previously. It is interesting that the earliest symptoms associated with the acromegaly in this latter patient were of temporo-mandibular joint disturbance, probably the result of renewed bone growth.

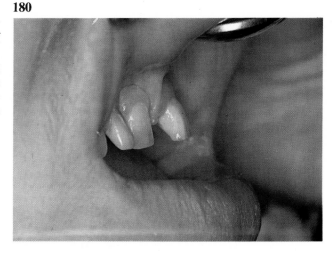

Leukoplakia and related lesions

The term leukoplakia ('white patch') is an entirely descriptive one, and it was used previously to include a wide range of white lesions of the oral mucosa. However, it is a term now used in a restricted manner according to the definition proposed by Pindborg: 'a white patch on the oral mucosa which cannot be wiped off and is not susceptible to any other clinical diagnosis'. In this way a large range of white lesions, (such as those of lichen planus) are excluded from this precise definition (see figure **84**).

Leukoplakia has for long been considered as an essentially pre-malignant condition. With the adoption of Pindborg's definition which contains no element of prognosis or histological implications, this interpretation can no longer be accepted as being true in all cases or, even, in the majority of cases. The term leukoplakia remains an entirely clinical one and is generally accepted as implying a lesion of non-specific histology, with a variable behaviour pattern but with an unpredictable (but statistically assessable) tendency to malignant transformation.

A number of lesions have been recognised as having a close relationship with leukoplakia and these are also illustrated in the present section.

181

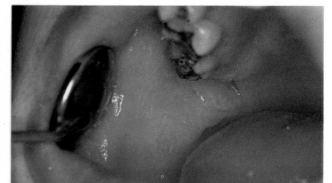

181 Leukoedema This is the term used to describe a condition in which the oral mucosa and, in particular, the buccal mucosa, presents with a grey appearance, rather as if a superficial film were lying on the mucosa itself. Opinions vary about this condition – some consider it to be a normal finding while others associate it with tobacco smoking. One reason for the extreme variability in the reported incidence of the condition in different surveys may well be the difficulty in its visualisation under certain artificial light sources. The patient illustrated was a cigarette smoker (30 daily) and, as is invariably the case, there were no symptoms attributable to the leukoedema.

182

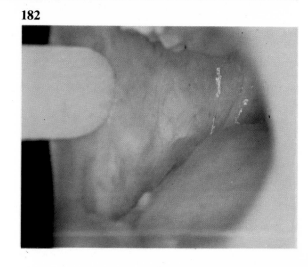

182 Preleukoplakia This is a term used to describe a diffuse white lesion of the mucosa, less dense and less marked than leukoplakia. It is considered that this marks a half-way stage in the production of leukoplakia. The patient illustrated is a 13 year-old boy from a family with a genetically determined tendency to oral leukoplakia associated with oesophageal carcinoma and tylosis (palmar-plantar hyperkeratosis). In these patients the preleukoplakias of childhood are eventually replaced by leukoplakias in adult life.

183 Leukoplakia of tongue The lesion shown is an homogenous leukoplakia in a male patient of 83 years.

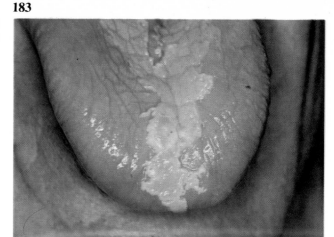

184 Leukoplakia of commissures and buccal mucosa This homogenous leukoplakia, in a characteristic site, showed few signs of epithelial atypia on biopsy. The patient smoked 30 cigarettes daily but there was no absolute evidence of a causal relationship.

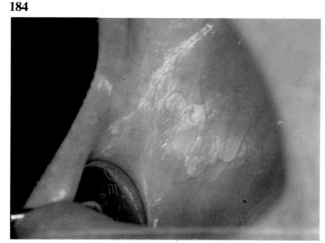

185 'Ebbing tide' leukoplakia This lesion of the floor-of-mouth and tongue shows the so-called 'ebbing tide' pattern. It was formerly thought a lesion such as this was of developmental origin and with no premalignant potential but it is now realised that the behaviour is similar to that of other homogenous leukoplakias.

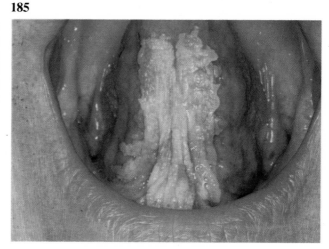

186 Leukoplakia of floor-of-mouth This widespread leukoplakia of the alveolar mucosa and floor-of-mouth showed marked epithelial atypia on biopsy. Surgical excision was necessary. The rather dense texture and irregular surface is seen often, though not invariably, in the more histologically aggressive lesions. Assessment of premalignant potential is possible only after histological study – clinical assessment alone is unreliable.

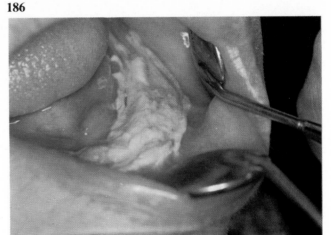

187 Speckled leukoplakia In speckled leuko-plakia, white areas alternate with areas of atrophic red epithelium. These lesions are frequently associated with candidal infection and have a much higher incidence of malignant transformation than homogenous leukoplakias. All leukoplakias with a recognisable candidal infiltration of the epithelium, and all those presenting clinically associated areas of atrophic red epithelium (erythroplakia) must be treated with suspicion as having a relatively high chance of malignant change.

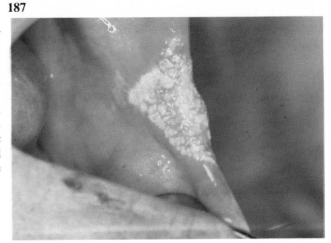

188 Candidal leukoplakia In this section, stained with periodic acid – Schiff reagent, the candidal pseudo-hyphae are seen penetrating the outer layers of the epithelium. This is a section of the lesion shown in figure **190**.

189 Candidal leukoplakia This illustrates the development of early leukoplakias in areas of persistent superficial candidal infection. The patient had suffered from angular cheilitis for many years, but the white lesions were of recent origin.

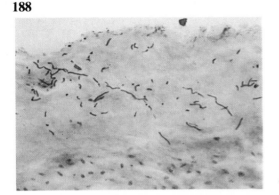

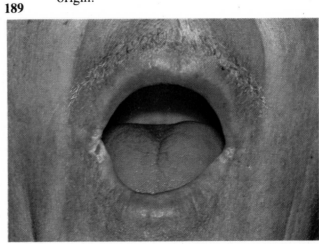

(See also figure **143**.)

190, 191, 192 Leukoplakia associated with cigarette smoking The patient illustrated was a heavy cigarette smoker (50 daily). The lesion shown in figure **190** was found on biopsy to have epithelial atypia and candidal infiltration of the epithelium. The smoking habit was discontinued and antifungal therapy applied. This resulted in clinical regression of the lesion within three months (figure **191**). One year later, the lesion presented with areas of erythroplakia (figure **192**) and biopsy showed marked epithelial atypia without candidal involvement. The recurrence of lesions following the removal of apparent aetiological factors is well documented.

190

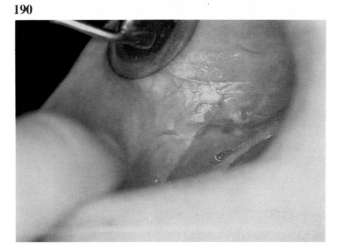

191 Regression of the lesion shown in figure **190** after 3 months without the use of tobacco.

191

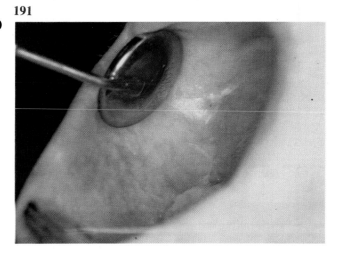

192 Recurrence of the lesion of figures **190** and **191** after one year.

192

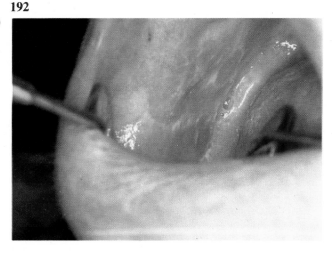

193 Leukoplakia of lower lip The lesion illustrated is a typical leukoplakia of the lower lip – somewhat thickened and hyperplastic in appearance. These lesions have a reputation for a high rate of malignant transformation ('the lip at risk') and it is suggested that exposure to sunlight may contribute to this.

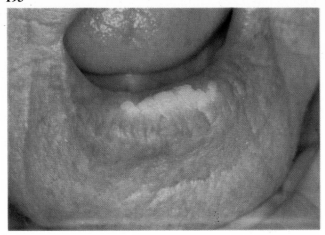

194 Leukoplakia associated with syphilis Syphilitic leukoplakia of the tongue is a classic manifestation of the late stages of the disease. It is now rarely seen in European conditions. The rate of malignant transformation is high, and it has been suggested that the behaviour of the lesions is a consequence of the immuno-suppression which occurs in tertiary syphilis.

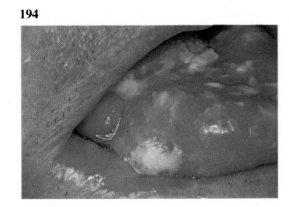

195 Leukoplakia of the palate This patchy leukoplakia of the palate was associated with similar lesions in other sites of the oral mucosa. Although there are some similarities in appearance this is not the typical 'smoker's palate' (see figure **196**).

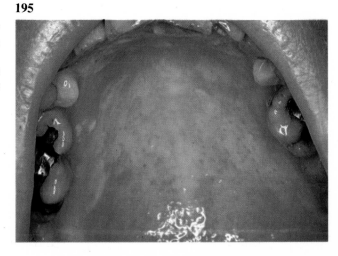

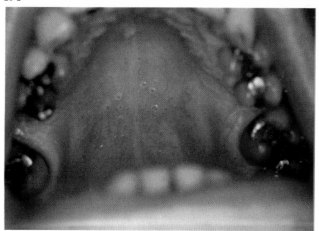

196 Smoker's keratosis of the palate 'Smoker's palate' occurs predominantly in pipe smokers, although from time to time it is seen in cigar and cigarette smokers. The characteristic feature is the enlargement of palatal mucous glands and the dilatation of their ducts to produce a central red spot. These stand in contrast to the generally white background of the palatal mucosa. There is often an intensification of the whiteness at the palatal gingival margins of the teeth. In European conditions of tobacco usage this is not considered to be a premalignant lesion.

197

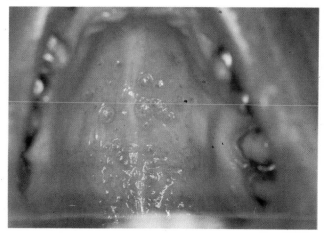

197 Papillomatosis of the palate A condition which may show superficial similarities to the smoker's keratosis of the palate is multiple papillomatosis. In this condition a number of small papillomas may be present though not specifically associated with the mucous glands. There are widely divergent views as to the significance of this condition – some consider it entirely benign while others prefer to treat it as a premalignant lesion.

198

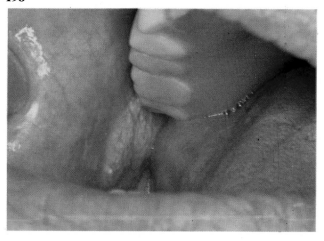

198 Frictional keratosis It is well known that prolonged frictional contact will induce changes in the patterns of keratinisation of the oral mucosa, although there is little agreement as to the actual mechanism for this. A typical clinical situation is illustrated here – repeated trauma produced by the rather sharp-edged denture has led to the production of a white patch on the buccal mucosa. Such lesions are usually hyperkeratinised (ortho- or para-) and there is little evidence that they have any marked tendency to malignant change.

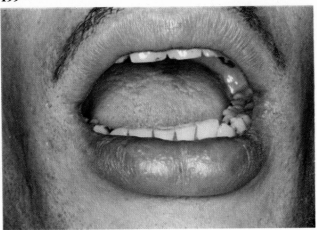

199, 200 Submucous fibrosis This is a condition which occurs virtually exclusively among inhabitants of India, Malaysia and nearby countries. Dense fibrous tissue is laid down in the submucosa leading to a binding down of the tongue and a restriction in mouth opening. This is followed by atrophic changes in the oral epithelium which takes on a marbled appearance. Although it is not known with certainty to be a premalignant condition, it is suggested that transformation of the affected epithelium to leukoplakia and then to carcinoma may frequently occur. The cause of this condition is not known – hypersensitivity to chillies and other spices has been suggested but the evidence is by no means conclusive.

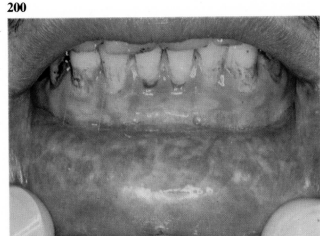

200 This illustrates the marbled appearance of the labial mucosa in submucous fibrosis.

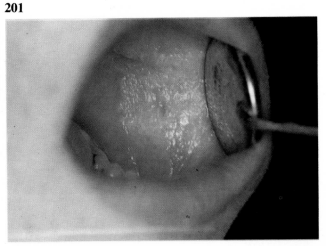

201 Cheek Chewing The lesion shown here is typical of those resulting from a cheek chewing habit. There are eroded areas and loose tags of partially detached mucous membrane, all lying within range of the occlusal plane of the teeth involved.

202 Plummer-Vinson syndrome In this syndrome (also known as the Patterson-Brown-Kelly syndrome), there is an association between iron deficiency anaemia and dysphagia, often associated with the presence of an oesophageal web. There is often atrophy of the lingual papillae and, as in this case, there may be areas of leukoplakia present on the tongue. These leukoplakias have a sinister reputation for malignant transformation.

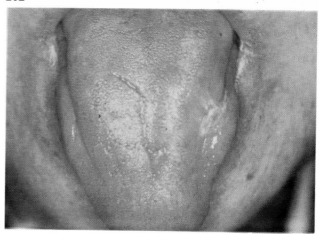

203

203 Radiation changes in buccal mucosa This is an illustration of the buccal mucosa of a patient who had undergone high voltage radiation therapy for a reticulum cell sarcoma in the cheek. The mucosa appears atrophic with patchy erythematous areas and numerous dilated capillaries.

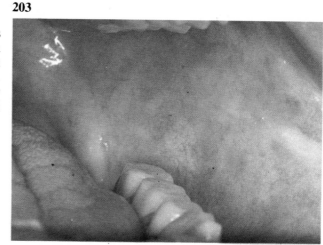

204

204 Fordyce's spots This condition is included in the present section although it represents a completely normal situation. Fordyce's spots are the sebaceous glands of the oral mucosa which vary considerably from patient to patient in number, distribution and prominence. During episodes of mild stomatitis (as, for instance, during the course of the common cold) the glands may come into more than usual prominence. Their greatest significance, however, is the fact that they are frequently mistaken for pathological structures and so are of importance in differential diagnosis.

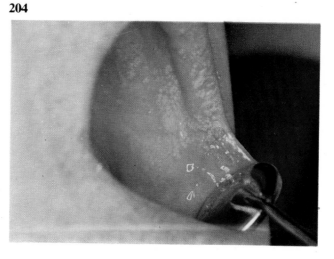

Inflammatory overgrowths and neoplasms

There is a wide range of inflammatory lesions of the oral mucosa which occur as a response to irritation or infection. These may appear in clinically distinguishable typical forms but occasionally this is not so and final diagnosis depends on histological assessment.

The term epulis (plural: epulides) has the literal meaning of a lump on the gum. It is used to describe discrete lesions produced as a result of irritation or inflammatory change on the gingival margin. It has no specific histological connotations.

A wide variety of neoplasms, both benign and malignant, primary or secondary, may appear in the oral cavity. Some of these are illustrated here in typical form, but atypical forms may also present and may lead to false diagnosis unless histological investigation is carried out. Of these lesions, oral carcinoma is by far the most significant in terms of incidence, distribution and subsequent effects.

205

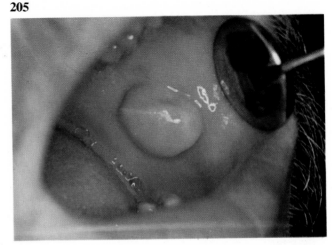

205, 206 Fibro-epithelial polyp This lesion consists essentially of scar tissue produced as a response to trauma. Thus, it is most often seen in sites adjacent to the occlusal plane. Occasionally, however, other locations may be involved.

206

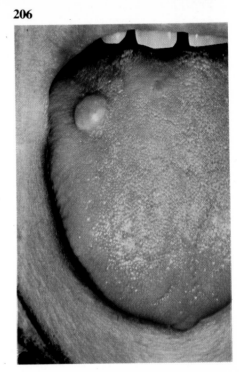

206 This illustration is of a fibro-epithelial polyp on the dorsum of the tongue – an unusual site.

207 Denture granuloma The denture granuloma is a similar lesion to the fibro-epithelial polyp, modified by the morphology of the tissues and by the nature of the irritant (in this case the flange of a denture). As in the case of the fibro-epithelial polyp, the denture granuloma is considered to be an entirely benign lesion.

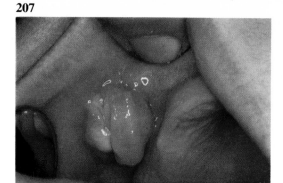

208 Fibrous epulis The fibrous epulis, essentially consisting of mature granulation tissue, grows slowly and often causes the patient little trouble. Its precise colour and texture depends on the degree of maturity of the lesion and on the presence or absence of secondary inflammatory changes. For some not very clear reason there is a preponderance of female patients among those with an epulis (4:1).

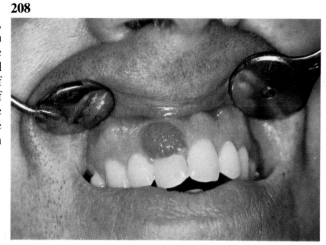

209 Fibrous epulis In some patients, neglect of the symptom-free lesion may lead to the production of unusually large epulides as in the illustration. These are practically always traumatised, hence secondarily ulcerated as in the present instance. There seems to be little, if any, premalignant potential in these lesions although it must be remembered that very occasionally true neoplasms (either primary or secondary) may appear in this site.

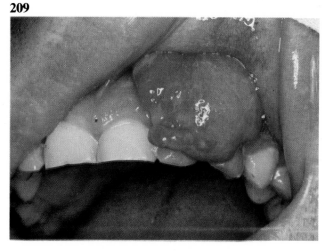

210 Pyogenic granuloma This is a variant of the fibrous epulis in which the granulation tissue remains vascular and immature. It has, therefore, a higher cellular content and, also, a higher vascular content than the more common fibrous epulis.

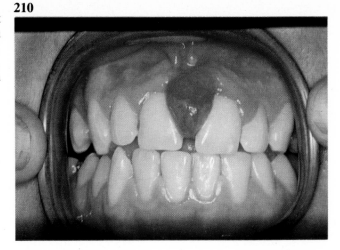

211 Giant cell epulis In the giant cell epulis the granulation tissue of which the lesion is formed includes an osteogenic component. On histological examination the tissue is seen to contain a variable number of multinucleated giant cells. This is particularly so in the immature forms of the lesion. In the more established lesions bone formation may occur. Giant cell epulides occur most frequently in children of either sex or in women of child-bearing age. Male adults are rarely affected.

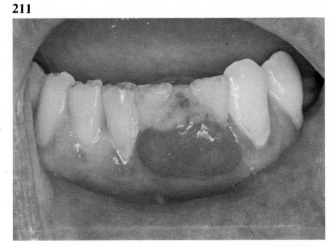

212 Papilloma A papilloma is not an inflammatory overgrowth but is a true benign epithelial neoplasm. This illustration is of such a lesion on the ventral surface of the tongue, but it is commonly found at the junction of the hard and soft palate. Oral papillomas do not have the tendency to malignant transformation shown by those in the lower gut.

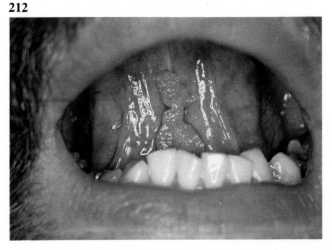

213 Papilloma of palate below a denture
When a papilloma grows below the fitting surface
of an upper denture it often assumes a flattened
disc-like form which is compressed into a
depression in the palatal mucosa. The pedicle
is developed into a small hinge about which the
flap-like lesion may be displaced downwards.
In their undisplaced position these lesions may
be easily missed on cursory examination.

213

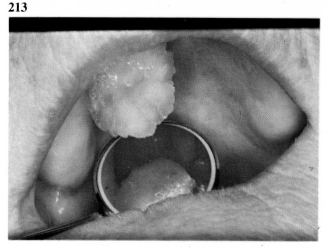

214

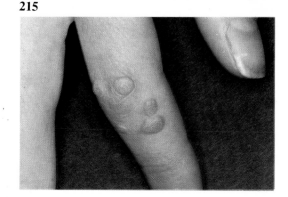

215

214, 215 Viral warts These are papilloma-like lesions which occur in response to infection by a specific
virus. They most commonly occur on the hands and fingers and may be transmitted, as in this case, to the
oral mucosa or lips by biting or chewing on these lesions. Unlike true papillomas, viral warts have a limited
life and spontaneous resolution may be expected within a year.

216 Haemangioma of tongue Angiomatous
lesions, either of the blood vessels or of the
lymphatic vessels, may occur anywhere in the
oral mucosa and may behave in an almost static
manner or may, as in the present instance, show
evidence of significant enlargement. Even so it
is by no means certain that these lesions
represent true neoplasms – it may well be that
they are, in fact, hamartomas undergoing changes
in the vascular dynamics (see figure **154**).

216

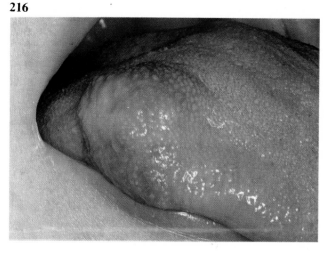

217 Lymphangioma of tongue The lymphangioma resembles the haemangioma in that there are doubts as to whether it represents a true neoplasm or a developmental abnormality. The present lesion in a nine year-old boy is somewhat unusual in its relatively dense whiteness. Often the lesion is more diffuse and nodular, resembling the lesion shown in figure **218**. However, this lesion is characteristic both in its site (most oral lymphangiomas are found on the tongue) and in the low age at which it has been discovered in the patient.

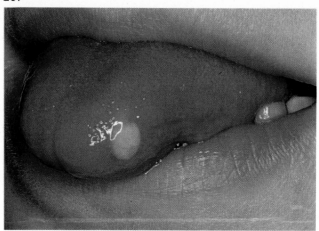

218 Angioma of the tongue The rather nodular appearance of the tongue is often described as characteristic of the lymphangioma. In this instance, the lesion was mixed, there being components which were clearly of a haemangiomatous nature and others which were felt to be lymphangiomatous.

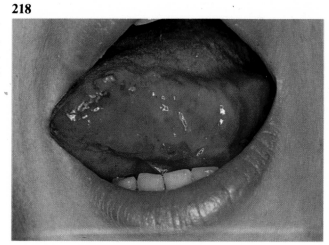

219 Salivary gland tumour of palate Salivary tumours of various kinds occur quite frequently in the mouth and, in particular, at the junction of the hard and soft palates where a high concentration of mucous glands is normally present. The majority of these neoplasms are pleomorphic adenomas but more aggressive lesions, such as adenocystic carcinomas, may have precisely similar clinical characteristics, at least in the early stages. The lesion illustrated here, a pleomorphic adenoma, shows the relatively symptom-free nature of many of these lesions and also their slow-growing behaviour. In this instance the apparently static palatal swelling had been mistaken for a lesion of no significance and the denture constructed so as to avoid it. The growth over several years had been apparently minimal.

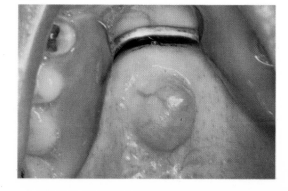

220 Salivary gland tumour of palate In this example of a pleomorphic adenoma of the palate, a much more aggressive growth picture is demonstrated. This lesion, filling the vault of the palate, had been present for less than a year and, although histologically non-malignant, it was in fact infiltrating the palatal bone. Such unpredictable behaviour is characteristic of the whole group of salivary tumours which should always be treated with suspicion, whatever their apparent clinical characteristics.

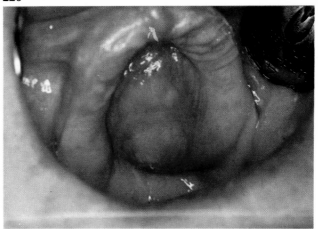

221 Carcinoma of buccal mucosa This is a relatively early and quite painless lesion occurring in the site from which a leukoplakia had been excised some time previously.

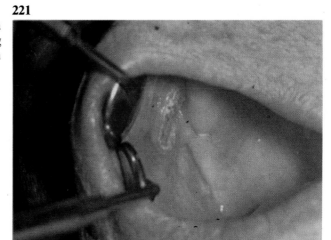

222 Carcinoma of floor-of-mouth In this lesion there is evident ulceration of the floor-of-mouth extending on to the ventral surface of the tongue and on to the alveolar ridge. White leukoplakia-like areas can be seen lying peripherally to the ulcerated lesion. In this instance the alveolar bone was invaded by the neoplasm.

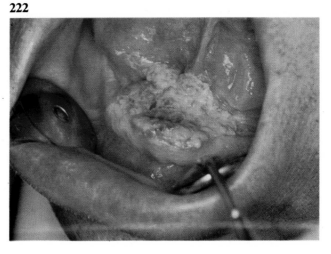

223 Carcinoma of alveolar mucosa In this advanced lesion there is gross ulceration of the mandibular alveolar mucosa with extension to the floor-of-mouth and buccal mucosa. There was advanced bone destruction and marked involvement of the cervical lymph nodes.

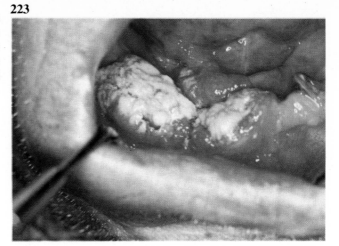

224 Carcinoma of alveolar mucosa This is a proliferative lesion extending to the buccal mucosa and the floor-of-mouth. In this case ulceration is minimal and the lesion had been mistaken for a denture granuloma.

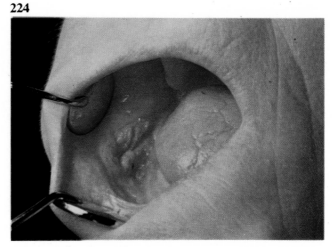

225 Carcinoma of palatal mucosa This lesion was primary to the palatal mucous membrane.

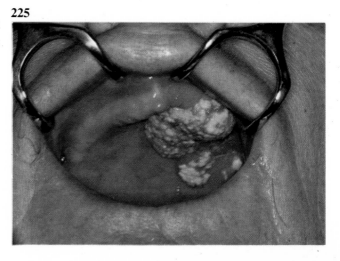

226 Carcinoma of floor-of-mouth This lesion of the floor-of-mouth with an extension on to the alveolar mucosa had not progressed sufficiently, at this stage, to cause radiographically detectable bone loss.

226

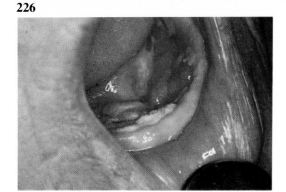

227 Carcinoma of the alveolar mucosa This lesion, in contrast to that of figure **226**, was associated with gross destruction of the underlying mandible.

227

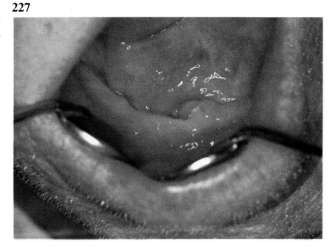

228 Widespread carcinoma of oral mucosa This illustrates a situation in which there is widespread malignant change over the epithelium of virtually the whole oral cavity. In such cases it is difficult to determine whether this represents transformation of a pre-existing leukoplakia or whether the lesion has arisen over a wide field *ab initio*. It would appear, however, that some intrinsic lack of stability of the oral epithelium is involved.

228

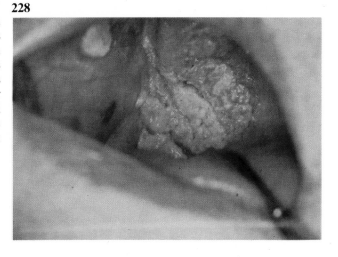

229 Carcinoma of the lip This represents an apparently special case in that the prognosis is considerably better than that of lesions within the oral cavity. Characteristically the patient was an elderly male and the lesion was on the lower lip. Equally characteristically, the lesion was quite painless and slow-growing, having been mistaken for a long-lasting herpetic lesion.

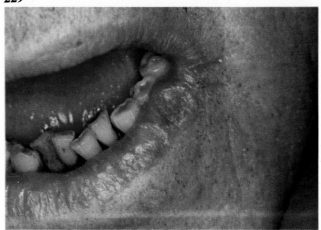

230 Malignant melanoma This illustration is of a patient with advanced primary intra-oral malignant melanoma. There were distant metastases, and a break-down of a lesion in the left buccal mucosa had led to spontaneous haemorrhage. The characteristic diffusely pigmented areas in the palate are evident.

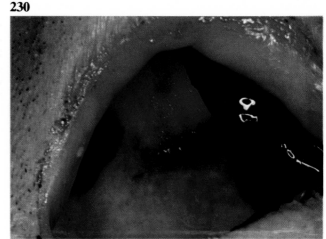

231 Inflammatory lesion simulating carcinoma This lesion is included to illustrate the possibility of mistaken clinical diagnosis in such instances. In this case a proliferative lesion was present with many of the characteristics of a carcinoma. Biopsy, however, showed this to be a secondarily infected denture granuloma.

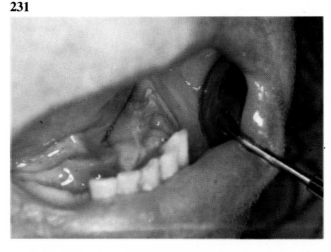

232 Osteosarcoma Although not strictly a lesion of the oral mucosa, this illustration is included in this section as a reminder of the fact that malignant lesions of the supporting bone may appear in the mouth. This lesion was an osteosarcoma of the maxilla in a young female patient, it having grown to the size illustrated without pain or any other marked symptoms.

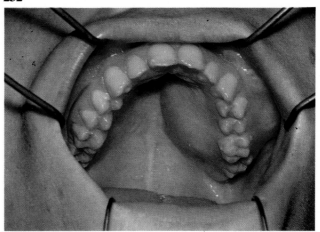

Salivary gland abnormalities

233

233 Mucous cyst (mucocele) Mucous cysts may be produced either as a result of mechanical trauma (mucous extravasation cyst) or by obstruction. In either case the clinical result is the same. These cysts are most commonly sited on the lower lip.

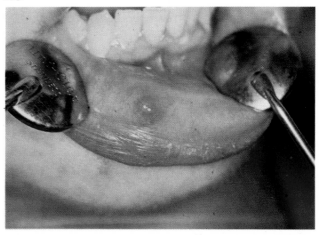

234

234 Ranula A ranula is a mucous cyst lying in the floor-of-mouth and arising from one of the salivary structures in this area.

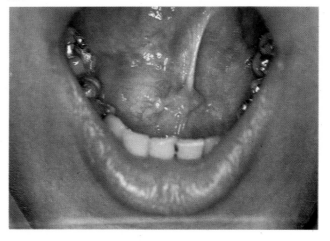

235, 236, 237, 238 Sjögren's syndrome This is a condition in which three factors are associated: dry mouth (xerostomia), lack of tear secretion leading to a keratoconjunctivitis (figure **236**), and the presence of an auto-immune disease – commonly rheumatoid arthritis. The presence of dry eyes and a dry mouth, in the absence of auto-immune disease, is usually referred to as sicca syndrome. The oral symptoms in Sjögren's syndrome, apart from the dryness of the mouth, consist of a thin and atrophic oral mucosa often together with a lobulated tongue (figure **235**).

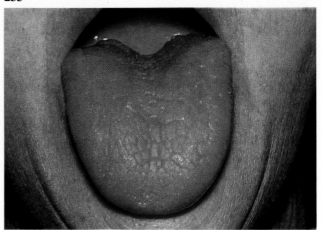

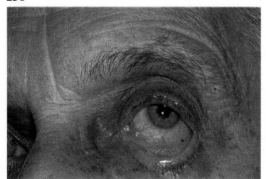

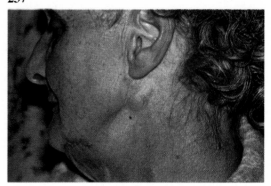

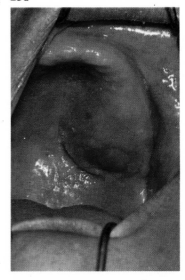

Swelling of major salivary glands (figure **237**) is an inconstant finding and swelling associated with minor salivary gland tissue is rare (figure **238**). The essential pathological process is the replacement of secreting salivary tissue by lymphoid tissue.

(See also figures **219**, **220**.)

Abnormalities of the teeth

The teeth are stable structures and play virtually no part in metabolic disease after their final calcification and eruption. It follows, therefore, that the teeth represent the condition of the patient at the time of calcification. In erupted teeth (and with the exception of caries) only those conditions which lead to loss of teeth substance – erosion, abrasion, attrition – significantly affect their appearance. However, extrinsic stains may be acquired, as may intrinsic coloration of individual teeth, usually as the result of trauma.

It is evidently necessary when considering the relationship of the oral tissues to generalised disease to recognise abnormalities of tooth structure, and representative examples of teeth modified by systemic abnormalities are illustrated here.

239, 240 Abnormalities of tooth eruption (cleido-cranial dysostosis) Teeth missing from their normal place in the dental arch could have been extracted, may be congenitally absent or, perhaps, be unerupted. In general terms partial anodontia is a purely local condition with no systemic manifestations. However, there exists a wide number of combined mesodermal-ectodermal dysplasias in which the teeth are either missing or of a relatively primitive form, or in which there are abnormalities in the eruption of the teeth. The present illustration is of a 20 year-old female in which the apparent abnormality was the retention of all deciduous teeth. In fact, this does not represent the absence of permanent teeth but, on the contrary, the presence of many supernumerary teeth which, together with teeth of the normal series, remain unerupted. In cleido-cranial dysostosis, this dental abnormality is associated with defects in membrane bone formation which, in their turn, lead to bossing of the frontal bones and a deficiency in calcification or even complete absence of the clavicles. There are many such conditions jointly affecting bones and teeth – this is probably the best known.

239

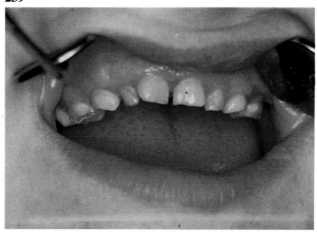

240

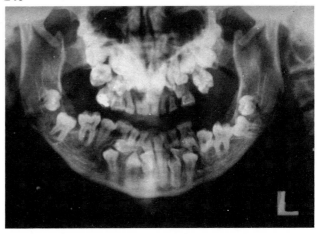

241 Attrition and abrasion Attrition is the wearing away of teeth by contact with other teeth. Abrasion is the term used to describe wear resulting from contact with some foreign body such as a tooth-brush. Both are markedly present in this patient. The orange appearance of the exposed dentine is due to tobacco staining and there is leukoedema of the mucosae.

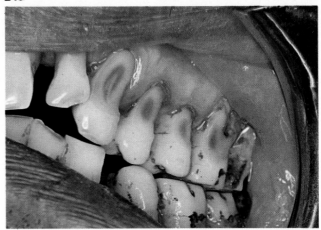

242 Erosion Erosion is the loss of dental tissues by solution in acids. Although formerly acid sprays produced in industrial processes were often implicated, the most common present-day cause of erosion is the use of acid drinks. Some medicines with an acid pH will naturally have the same effect, as may regular regurgitation of stomach acid.

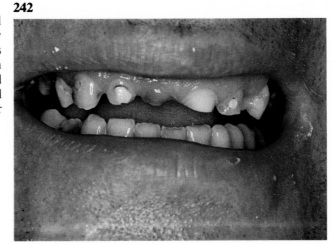

243 Amelogenesis imperfecta A deficiency of the enamel may result from generalised disease during the formation of the teeth or may be apparently spontaneous and, as in amelogenesis imperfecta, genetically determined. Two components may be recognised in amelogenesis imperfecta. The first of these, illustrated here, represents lack of adequate calcification of the enamel matrix – the enamel can be seen flaking away from the dentine. In other patients the enamel seems to be relatively well calcified but deficient in thickness or in structure. There is probably no absolutely clear distinction between these two forms. Amelogenesis imperfecta is only rarely associated with any generalised disease process.

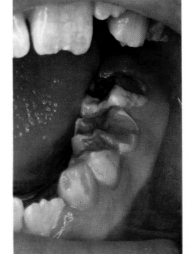

244 Enamel hypoplasia This illustrates the typical situation in which severe febrile illness occurred at the time of initial calcification of the upper cental incisors (within the first year of life).

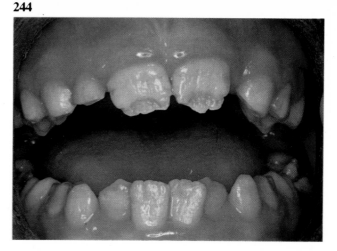

245 Enamel hypoplasia – fluorosis The brown pitting and staining seen in these teeth are characteristic of fluorosis. In this instance, the patient was born and spent his early childhood in a Mediterranean area of extremely high natural fluoride content in the drinking water.

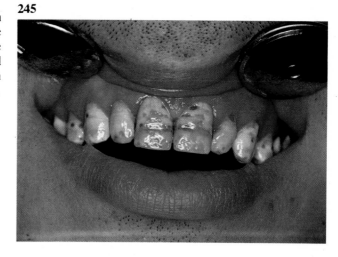

246 Dentinogenesis imperfecta In this condition the dentine is poorly formed and the teeth have a peculiarly opalescent appearance which leads to the term 'hereditary opalescent dentine'. This is often a genetically determined condition and may be associated with osteogenesis imperfecta. Members of families in which these conditions are associated may show only the abnormal dentine, without fragility of the bones, but in these circumstances they often show the blue sclera typical of osteogenesis imperfecta (figure **247**).

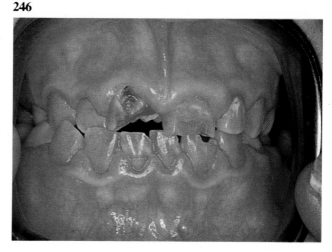

247 Osteogenesis imperfecta This patient was a member of a family all of whom showed dentinogenesis imperfecta, varying degrees of osteogenesis imperfecta, and blue sclera.

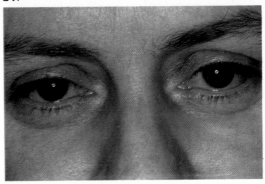
247

248 Hypoplasia due to calcium malabsorption In general, nutritional factors play very little rôle in the production of abnormalities of dental tissue. In this rare case, there was a major abnormality of calcium absorption with consequent deficiency in the dental tissues as well as in the bones. It should be emphasised that such aetiological factors are extremely rare.

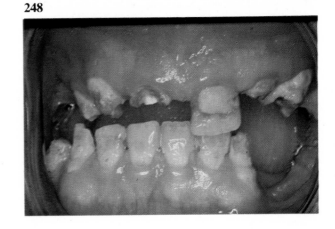
248

249, 250, 251, 252, 253 Tetracycline staining When tetracyclines are administered during the period of tooth formation, staining of the dentine and enamel may occur. The colours produced are variable as is the intensity of the staining. In figure **249** there is diffuse yellow staining which is not associated with any evident hypoplasia of the tooth substance. In figures

250, 251, 252 variable degrees of hypoplasia are present but these are probably dependent more on the general disease process for which the tetracyclines were administered than on the effect of the tetracycline itself.

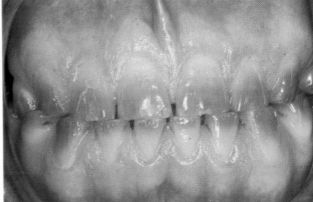
249

250 A boy with a renal transplant following renal failure due to nephrotic syndrome.

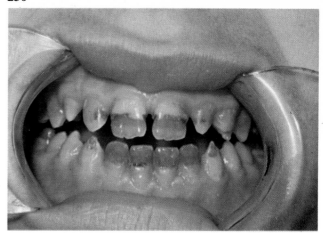

251 This marked tetracycline staining is in the patient with agranulocytosis illustrated in figure **149**.

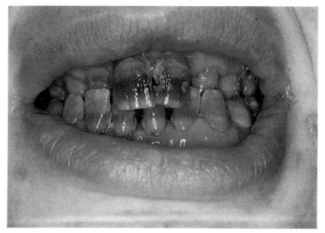

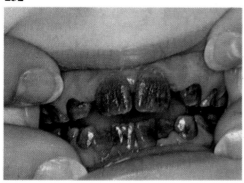

252 The tetracycline had been given prophylactically to this patient with cystic fibrosis.

253 In this patient tetracycline staining of the deciduous teeth is associated with enamel hypoplasia in the permanent teeth.

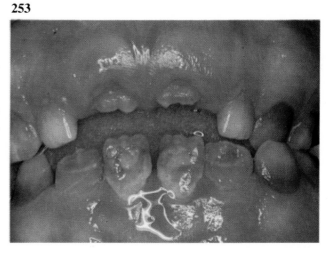

254 Neonatal jaundice In this young patient the coloration of the teeth is due to pigment deposited as a result of neonatal jaundice. There is evidently some degree of hypoplasia associated with the coloration.

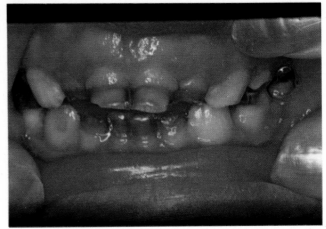

(See also figures **28, 29, 114**.)

Lesions of bone

A wide range of lesions of bone may be seen in and around the jaws but the vast majority of these are of inflammatory origin (for example, dental cysts) or relatively simple bone overgrowths and exostoses. There are, however, two dystrophic conditions of bone which are seen from time to time in the jaws. These are Paget's disease and fibrous dysplasia. Other dystrophic or metabolic bone diseases are extremely rare, although developmental abnormalities of form are less so.

255 Torus mandibularis This is an example of a simple bony outgrowth in a characteristic site. Other similar lesions are often seen in the midline of the hard palate.

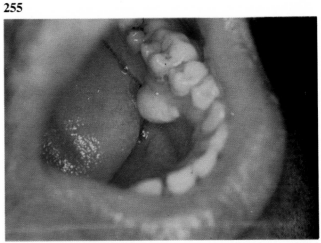

256, 257 Fibrous dysplasia Monostotic fibrous dysplasia is a fairly common disease of the jaws in which there is partial replacement of the normal bone by fibrous tissue. As the name implies this occurs usually as an isolated lesion, most commonly, as in this instance, unilaterally in the maxilla. There is no widespread biochemical change as measured by variations in blood chemistry.

256

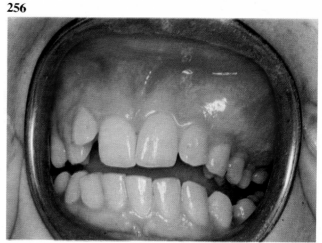

257 The radiograph of the patient shown in figure **256** shows obliteration of the maxillary sinus by the bone growth of fibrous dysplasia.

257

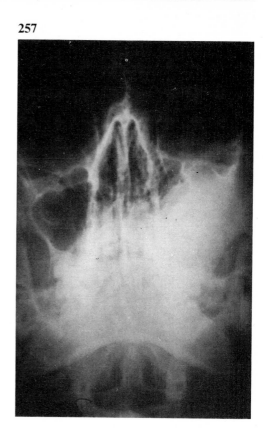

258, 259, 260 Polystotic fibrous dysplasia (Allbright's syndrome) In contrast to monostotic fibrous dysplasia this is a condition which may be widespread throughout the skeleton, including the skull and jaws. Apart from the replacement of normal bone architecture by fibrous tissue, there are widespread endocrine changes reflected in precocious puberty and hyperpigmentation of skin. The illustrations are of an eight year-old boy with widespread skeletal involvement.

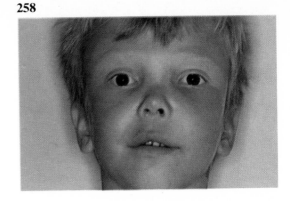

259 This shows the patchy hyperpigmentation of the skin.

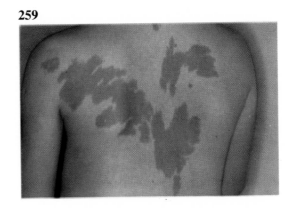

260 The radiograph of the skull shows the gross distortion of bone structure. There were equivalent changes in other bones.

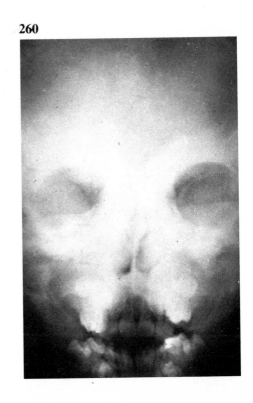

261

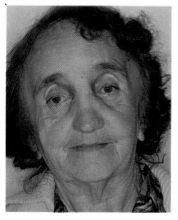

262

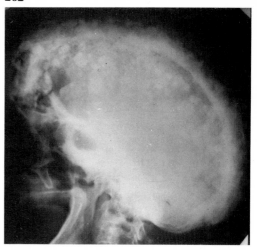

261, 262   Paget's disease   Paget's disease is a common condition in elderly patients but in most cases it is symptom-free and is not discovered except as an incidental finding. In this condition there is concurrent resorption of bone and the laying down of other abnormal bone. This process not infrequently is most active in and about the facial bones and skull and the first complaint of the patient may be that previously well-fitting dentures have apparently become too small. The distortion of the skull is evident in the patient shown.

263, 264   Paget's disease of maxilla   In this patient, the areas of Pagetoid bone were relatively circumscribed to two dense masses in the maxilla. Histological study and blood chemistry showed these to be localised lesions of Paget's disease.

263

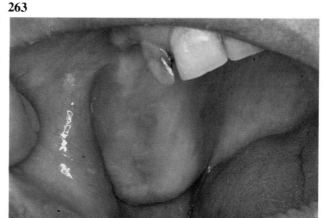

264   The radiograph of the patient shown in figure **263** demonstrates the two dense masses of abnormal bone in the maxillae.

264

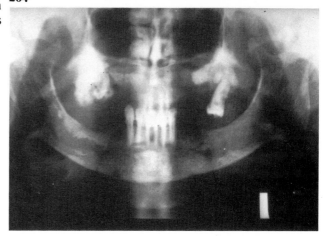

(See also figures **232, 239**.)

Notes on the diagnostic features
of some groups of common conditions

RECURRENT ORAL ULCERATION

1. **Minor aphthous ulceration** (figures **39–42**) 1–6 ulcers at a time.
   Size variable – usually 2–10mm diameter.
   Duration short – usually 10 days; variable free period.
   Site – not throat or palate. Healing without scars.

2. **Major aphthous ulceration** (figures **44–46**) Variable number of predominantly large ulcers.
   Duration long – may be months.
   Site – anywhere on oral mucosa and oro-pharynx. Healing with scar formation.

3. **Herpetiform ulceration** (figures **47–48**) Many small but painful ulcers.
   Duration variable – 1–2 weeks usual.
   Site – floor-of-mouth, lateral margin and tip of tongue most common. Healing without scars.

Associated lesions – genital, eye, or skin lesions. Occasional C.N.S., joint and vascular lesions (= Behçet's syndrome).

Associated conditions – coeliac disease, anaemias, nutritional disturbances.

Diagnosis – mainly by clinical features. Supplementary investigations – haematology screen, jejunal biopsy.

Important differential diagnoses
Carcinoma (from major aphthous ulcer)
Viral infections (from herpetiform ulceration)
Erosive lichen planus
Traumatic ulcer.

BULLOUS AND VESICULAR LESIONS

(a) *Acute*

1. **Primary herpes** (figures **1–8**) Vesicles on whole of oral mucosa – may be some on lips and perioral skin.
   Vesicles rapidly break down to form ulcers.
   Marked gingivitis – especially in children.
   Malaise and fever often precedes vesicles.
   A non-recurrent condition – often following contact with chronic herpetic lesion.
   Young children and young adults commonly affected.

Diagnosis – clinical, epithelial smears, viral growth, antibody titre studies, electron microscopy.

Important differential diagnosis
In adults – from erythema multiforme
In children – from acute leukaemia.

2. **Erythema multiforme** (figures **116–120**) Vesicles on whole of oral mucosa – often on lower lip. Vesicles rapidly break down to form ulcers with crusting lip.
A recurrent condition. Attacks may be precipitated by a variety of factors – infection, drugs etc.
Young adults commonly affected.

Associated lesions (figures **122, 123**) – 'target' lesions of skin; genital or eye inflammation.

Diagnosis – clinical. Negative results of tests for viral origin.

(b) *Chronic or Subacute*

1. **Pemphigus** (figures **100–104**) Bullae rapidly breaking down to form erosions. Oral mucosa, other mucous membranes and skin affected. Half of all cases begin in mouth.
Predominantly 40–60-year-olds.
Jewish patients have high incidence. Progressive disease.

Diagnosis – histology, immunological (immunofluorescence) cytology of bulla fluid.

2. **Pemphigoid** (figures **107–108**) Relatively firm bullae. Oral mucosa affected in only 20 per cent of patients.
60 years +. No racial prevalence. Less rapidly progressive than pemphigus, but recurrent.

Diagnosis – as pemphigus.

3. **Benign mucous membrane pemphigoid** (figure **111**) Bullae of mucous membrane rupturing and healing with scar formation. Affects restricted areas especially soft palate and conjunctivae. Predominantly female patients (2:1) aged 60 years +. No racial prevalence. Relatively static but may cause blindness.

Diagnosis – as pemphigus.

4. **Bullous lichen planus** (figure **98**) A relatively rare variant of lichen planus – may be a transient stage. Fragile bullae rapidly breaking down to form erosions. Usually associated areas of non-bullous lichen planus.

Associated lesions – of skin in some patients.

Diagnosis – from histology.

Important differential diagnosis
Pemphigus from others.

See also:
    Dermatitis herpetiformis (figure **112**)
    Epidermolysis bullosa (figures **113–115**)

WHITE PATCHES OF THE ORAL MUCOSA

1. **Traumatic keratosis** (figure **198**) Identified by relationship to irritant (e.g. broken tooth). May be associated with cheek or lip chewing habits. Possibly associated ulceration.

Diagnosis – clinical.

2. **Chemical burns** (figure **161**) Usually due to aspirin and near a carious tooth. Acute onset. Thickened dense white patch – may be painful.

Diagnosis – from history (including toothache).

3. **Leukoplakia** (figures **184–187**) Wide range of clinical presentations including variants: homogenous, speckled (figure **187**), erythroplakia (figure **192**).
Spontaneous or associated with tobacco (figures **190–192**) or candidal infection (figures **188–189**).

Associated conditions – rarely, late syphilis, iron deficiency (figures **143, 194, 202**).

Diagnosis – histology essential.

Important differential diagnoses
From carcinoma, lichen planus.

4. **Carcinoma** (figure **228**) May present as a white patch initially.

Diagnosis – histology essential.

5. **Lichen planus** (figures **84–85**) May present as confluent white lesions (figures **84–85**) as well as reticulated or erosive forms (see variants figures **82–99**).

Associated lesions – of skin in some patients (figures **79–81**); not necessarily at the same time.

Associated conditions – maturity onset diabetes mellitus (as yet uncertain).

Diagnosis – histology to confirm clinical.

Important differential diagnosis
From acute pseudomembranous candidiasis (thrush) (figure **14**).

All white patches should be biopsied for accurate diagnosis.

See also:
   Chronic discoid lupus (figure **125**)
   Smoker's keratosis of palate (figure **196**)

SORE AND DEPAPILLATED TONGUE

1. **Traumatic** (figure **43**) Often associated with habits. Commonly at the tip or at the root of the tongue. May or may not be an evident irritant (e.g. broken tooth).

Diagnosis – clinical.

2. **Geographic tongue (erythema migrans)** (figures **66–69**) Characteristic appearance and history. Irritated by strongly flavoured foods.

Diagnosis – clinical.

3. **Sore tongue in haematological abnormalities** (figures **70, 71, 137–141**) May be depapillated, red, ulcerated, or apparently normal in appearance. May be changes in taste sensation.

Associated lesions – diffuse stomatitis, angular cheilitis, candidiasis etc.

Associated conditions – wide range of anaemias, latent anaemias and nutritional deficiencies.

Diagnosis – full blood screening followed by haematology work up.

4. **Sjögren's syndrome** (figure **72**) Tongue dry and lightly fissured. Oral mucosa in general dry and shiny.

Associated lesions – may be dry eyes, swollen salivary glands.

Associated conditions – auto-immune diseases.

Diagnosis – tests of salivary flow functions, haematology, labial gland biopsy.

5. **Lichen planus** (figure **96**) – after re-epithelialisation of eroded areas.

Diagnosis – from history.

6. **Antibiotic sore tongue** (figure **73**) – atrophic candidiasis, red and painful tongue following course of antibiotics. (Usually tetracyclines)

Diagnosis – from history.

7. **Median glossitis** (figures **59–64**) Red patch in midline of tongue. Not necessarily painful.

Associated conditions – occasionally anaemias.

Diagnosis – clinical, confirmed by histology.

Important differential diagnosis
From erythroplakia or carcinoma.

PIGMENTATION OF THE ORAL MUCOSA

1. **Amalgam tattoo** (figure **178**) Discrete areas usually on or near gingivae. Long history.

Diagnosis – clinical. Radiography, histology.

2. **Racial pigmentation** (figure **177**) Diffuse, most intense at gingivae. Can occur in all races.

3. **Endocrine (Addison's disease)** (figure **176**) Patchy melanotic area on buccal mucosa and palate.

Associated lesions – pigmentation of skin, candidiasis.

Associated conditions – generalised malaise, weight loss, hypotension.

Diagnosis – endocrinological.

4. **Benign melanoma and naevae**
   Relatively rare in oral cavity compared to skin. Associated with gut pathology in Peutz-Jegher's syndrome (figures **134–135**).

Diagnosis – by biopsy excision, if in doubt of history.

5. **Malignant melanoma** (figure **230**) Aggressive neoplasm.
   May be diffuse or papular.
   May be amelanotic.

Diagnosis – if suspected, by excision biopsy with wide margins.

6. **Drug-induced pigmentation** Heavy metals now rarely involved. Antimalarials (a greyish coloration of buccal and palatal mucosa) and oral contraceptives (darkening of labial mucosa) most commonly implicated.

Important differential diagnoses
Malignant melanoma from all other categories
From haemangioma, varices etc.

See also:
   Allbright's syndrome (figures **258–260**)

Note: melanotic pigmentation may accompany or follow some inflammatory lesions. It may occur in lichen planus and in some leukoplakias but is usually detected histologically – not clinically.

SOME COMMON INFECTIONS OF THE ORAL MUCOSA

1. **Acute ulcerative gingivitis (Vincent's gingivitis)** (figure 36) Bleeding, sore gingivae. Shallow ulcers on gingival papillae, spreading along margins.
Destruction of papillae.
Malaise, lymphadenitis, pyrexia and marked halitosis. Often recurrent.

Associated conditions – rarely: leukaemia or other debilitating condition may predispose (figure 37).

Diagnosis – mainly by clinical features, confirmation by direct bacteriological smear.

2. **Primary herpes** (figures 1–8) See under 'Bullous and Vesicular lesions'.

3. **Recurrent herpes** (figures 9, 10) Vesicular lesions on or near lips. Occasionally more widespread. Rupture of vesicles followed by crusting. Often recurrent in same site. Precipitated by sunlight, trauma or debilitating conditions.

Associated conditions – common cold, rarely leukaemia, pneumonia, during immuno-suppression.

Diagnosis – clinical. Confirmed by epithelial smears, viral growth.

4. **Candidiasis**

   (a) **Acute pseudomembranous candidiasis (thrush)** (figure 14) White patches overlying oral mucosa – wipe away leaving raw areas. Patches contain candidal hyphae.

Associated lesions – angular cheilitis, occasionally vaginal thrush.

Associated conditions – debilitating disease or immune deficiency (figure 175).

Diagnosis – clinical; by direct smear and culture. Investigations – e.g. haematology screen etc.

   (b) **Acute atrophic candidiasis** (figure 19) Fiery red mucosa. Epithelium thin and atrophic, no surface membrane. Associated with systemic steroid therapy or antibiotic treatment **(antibiotic sore tongue)** (figure 73).

Associated conditions – those requiring steroid or antibiotic therapy. Endocrine disturbances.

Diagnosis – clinical. Swabs may not yield many candida.

   (c) **Chronic atrophic candidiasis (denture sore mouth)** (figure 21) Red painless area under upper denture. May be granular and resemble hyperplastic tissue (figure 22). May also rarely appear in diffuse form (not associated with dentures) in endocrine disturbances (figures 20, 173, 174).

(c) **Chronic atrophic candidiasis** (continued)

Associated lesions – angular cheilitis.

Associated conditions – ill-fitting or old upper denture.

Diagnosis – clinical.

Note: angular cheilitis and median cracks of the lips may be infected either by candida or by staphylococci or both (figures **23, 30, 74**).

(d) **Chronic hyperplastic candidiasis (candidal leukoplakia)** (figure **189**) Appears as a leukoplakia, homogenous or speckled. Candida within the epithelium. The role of the candida is not known. High premalignant potential.

Diagnosis – histological (P.A.S. stain) (figure **188**).

See also:
   Less common infective conditions in section figures **1–38**.

Bibliography

Acute Ulcerative Gingivitis

BLAKE, G.C. (1968). The microbiology of acute ulcerative gingivitis with reference to the culture of oral trichomonads and spirochaetes. Proceedings of the Royal Society of Medicine, **61**, 131.

LEHNER, T. (1969). Immunoglobulin abnormalities in ulcerative gingivitis. British Dental Journal, **127**, 165

Bullous Lesions

COOKE, B.E.D. (1960). The diagnosis of bullous lesions affecting the oral mucosa. British Dental Journal, **109**, 83.

Cancrum Oris

EMSLIE, R.D. (1963). Cancrum Oris. Dental Practitioner, **13**, 481.

Candidiasis

HIGGS, J.M. and WELLS, R.S. (1973). Chronic mucocutaneous candidiasis: new approaches to treatment. British Journal of Dermatology, **89**, 179.

LEHNER, T. (1966). In WINNER, H.I. and HURLEY, R. Symposium on Candida Infections, 119-137. Churchill-Livingstone, Edinburgh, 1966.

Angular Cheilitis

MacFARLANE, T.W. and HELNARSKA, Sandra J. (1976). The microbiology of angular cheilitis. British Dental Journal, **140**, 403.

Candida Leukoplakia

CAWSON, R.A. (1966). Chronic oral candidosis and leukoplakia. Oral Surgery, Oral Medicine and Oral Pathology, **22**, 582.

CAWSON, R.A. and LEHNER, T. (1968). Chronic hyperplastic candidiasis – candidal leukoplakia. British Journal of Dermatology, **80**, 9.

Denture Sore Mouth

CAWSON, R.A. LEHNER, T. and NEILL, D.J. (1965). Symposium on Candidiasis. Dental Practitioner, **16**, 135.

Colitis (ulcerative)

McCARTHY, P. and SHKLAR, G. (1963). A syndrome of pyostomatitis vegetans and ulcerative colitis. Archives of Dermatology, **88**, 913.

Crohn's Disease (oral)

VERBOV, J. (1973). Crohn's disease with lip and mouth involvement. British Journal of Dermatology, **88**, 517.

Erythema Multiforme

BRITISH MEDICAL JOURNAL (Editorial) (1972). **1**, 63.

Geographic Tongue

BANOCZY, J., SZABO, L. and CSIBA, A. (1975). Migratory glossitis. Oral Surgery, Oral Medicine and Oral Pathology, **39**, 113.

Haematological Disturbances

WALKER, R.O., ROSE, M. (1965). Oral manifestations of haematological disorders. British Dental Journal, **23**, 286.

Anaemias etc

MASON, D.K., CHISHOLM, D.M., FERGUSON, M.M., HUNTER, I.P., LYELL, A. and STEPHEN, K.W. (1974). The Function and Organisation of an Oral Medicine Clinic. British Dental Journal, **136**, 232.

TYLDESLEY, W.R. (1975). Oral signs and symptoms in anaemias. British Dental Journal, **139**, 232.

Leukaemia

LYNCH, M.A. and SHIPP, I.I. (1967). Oral manifestations of Leukaemia: a post-diagnostic study *and* Initial oral manifestations of leukaemia. Journal American Dental Association, **75**, 1139 and 932.

Herpes Simplex and Zoster

JUEL-JENSEN, B.E. (1973). Herpes simplex and zoster. British Medical Journal, **1**, 406.

Bibliography

Leukoplakia and Carcinoma

BANOCZY, J. and CSIBA, A. (1972). Comparative study of the clinical picture and histopathologic structure of oral leukoplakia. Cancer, **29**, 1230.

BANOCZY, J. and SUGAR, L. (1972). Longitudinal studies in oral leukoplakia. Journal of Oral Pathology, **1**, 265.

BINNIE, W.H., CAWSON, R.A., HILL, G.B. and SOAPER, A.E. (1972). Oral Cancer in England and Wales. H.M.S.O., London.

CAWSON, R.A. (1969). Leukoplakia and oral cancer. Proceedings of the Royal Society of Medicine, **62**, 610–615.

PINDBORG, J.J., RENSTRUP, G., POULSEN, H.E. and SILVERMAN, S. (1963). Studies in oral leukoplakias V. Clinical and histologic signs of malignancy. Acta odontologica Scandinavia, **21**, 407.

TYLDESLEY, W.R. (1976). Oral Leukoplakia. Journal of the Royal College of Surgeons, Edinburgh, **21**, 148.

Lichen Planus

ANDREASEN, J.O. (1968). Oral lichen planus: a clinical evaluation of 115 cases. Oral Surgery, Oral Medicine and Oral Pathology, **25**, 31.

TYLDESLEY, W.R. (1974). Oral lichen planus. British Journal of Oral Surgery, **11**, 187.

Median Rhomboid Glossitis

COOKE, B.E. (1975). Median rhomboid glossitis: Candidiasis and not a developmental abnormality. British Journal of Dermatology, **93**, 399.

Melkersson-Rosenthal Syndrome

NALLY, F.F. (1970). Melkersson-Rosenthal syndrome. Oral Surgery, Oral Medicine and Oral Pathology, **29**, 694.

Recurrent Oral Ulceration

LEHNER, T. (1967). Autoimmunity and management of recurrent oral ulceration. British Dental Journal, **122**, 15.

LEHNER, T. (1969). Characterisation of mucosal antibodies in recurrent aphthous ulceration and Behçet's syndrome. Archives of Oral Biology, **14**, 843.

LEHNER, T. (1972). Immunological aspects of oral ulcers. Oral Surgery, Oral Medicine and Oral Pathology, **33**, 80.

Sjögren's Syndrome

CHISHOLM, D.M. and MASON, D.K. (1973). Sjögren's syndrome. British Dental Journal, **135**, 393.

Submucous Fibrosis

PINDBORG, J.J. and SIRSAT, S.M. (1966). Oral submucous fibrosis. Oral Surgery, Oral Medicine and Oral Pathology, **22**, 764.

Wegener's Granulomatosis

SCOTT, J. and FINCH, L.D. (1972). Wegener's granulomatosis presenting as gingivitis. Oral Surgery, Oral Medicine and Oral Pathology, **34**, 920.

Text-books and Collections

DOLBY, A.E. (Ed.) (1975). Oral Mucosa in Health and Disease. Blackwell, Oxford.

GORLIN, R.J. and PINDBORG, J.J. (1964). Syndromes of the Head and Neck. McGraw-Hill, New York.

JUEL-JENSEN, B.E. and MacCALLAM, F.D. (1972). Herpes Simplex, Varicella and Zoster. Heinemann, London.

MASON, D.K. and CHISHOLM, D.M. (1975). Salivary Glands in Health and Disease. W.B. Saunders, London.

PINDBORG, J.J. (1970). Pathology of the Dental Hard Tissues. Munsgaard, Copenhagen.

ROOKE, A.J., WILKINSON, D.S. and EBLING, F.J.G. (1973). Text-book of Dermatology, 2nd Edition, Blackwell, Oxford.

TYLDESLEY, W.R. (1978). Oral Diagnosis, 2nd Edition, Pergamon, Oxford.

WINNER, H.J. and HURLEY, R. (1966). Symposium on Candida Infections. Livingstone, Edinburgh.

INDEX

Figures in light type refer to page numbers
Figures in **bold** type refer to caption numbers

Index